T0362501

Challenging Current Wisdom in Hand Surgery

Editors

JIN BO TANG
GREY GIDDINS

HAND CLINICS

www.hand.theclinics.com

Consulting Editor
KEVIN C. CHUNG

August 2022 • Volume 38 • Number 3

ELSEVIER

1600 John F. Kennedy Boulevard • Suite 1800 • Philadelphia, Pennsylvania, 19103-2899

http://www.theclinics.com

HAND CLINICS Volume 38, Number 3
August 2022 ISSN 0749-0712, ISBN-13: 978-0-323-92017-9

Editor: Megan Ashdown
Developmental Editor: Hannah Almira Lopez

© **2022 Elsevier Inc. All rights reserved.**

This periodical and the individual contributions contained in it are protected under copyright by Elsevier, and the following terms and conditions apply to their use:

Photocopying

Single photocopies of single articles may be made for personal use as allowed by national copyright laws. Permission of the Publisher and payment of a fee is required for all other photocopying, including multiple or systematic copying, copying for advertising or promotional purposes, resale, and all forms of document delivery. Special rates are available for educational institutions that wish to make photocopies for non-profit educational classroom use. For information on how to seek permission visit www.elsevier.com/permissions or call: (+44) 1865 843830 (UK)/(+1) 215 239 3804 (USA).

Derivative Works

Subscribers may reproduce tables of contents or prepare lists of articles including abstracts for internal circulation within their institutions. Permission of the Publisher is required for resale or distribution outside the institution. Permission of the Publisher is required for all other derivative works, including compilations and translations (please consult www.elsevier.com/permissions).

Electronic Storage or Usage

Permission of the Publisher is required to store or use electronically any material contained in this periodical, including any article or part of an article (please consult www.elsevier.com/permissions). Except as outlined above, no part of this publication may be reproduced, stored in a retrieval system or transmitted in any form or by any means, electronic, mechanical, photocopying, recording or otherwise, without prior written permission of the Publisher.

Notice

No responsibility is assumed by the Publisher for any injury and/or damage to persons or property as a matter of products liability, negligence or otherwise, or from any use or operation of any methods, products, instructions or ideas contained in the material herein. Because of rapid advances in the medical sciences, in particular, independent verification of diagnoses and drug dosages should be made.

Although all advertising material is expected to conform to ethical (medical) standards, inclusion in this publication does not constitute a guarantee or endorsement of the quality or value of such product or of the claims made of it by its manufacturer.

Hand Clinics (ISSN 0749-0712) is published quarterly by Elsevier Inc., 360 Park Avenue South, New York, NY 10010-1710. Months of publication are February, May, August, and November. Business and Editorial Offices: 1600 John F. Kennedy Blvd., Ste. 1800, Philadelphia, PA 19103-2899. Customer Service Office: 3251 Riverport Lane, Maryland Heights, MO 63043. Periodicals postage paid at New York, NY and at additional mailing offices. Subscription price is $444.00 per year (domestic individuals), $1060.00 per year (domestic institutions), $100.00 per year (domestic students/residents), $506.00 per year (Canadian individuals), $1081.00 per year (Canadian institutions), $568.00 per year (international individuals), $1081.00 per year (international institutions), $256.00 (international students/residents), and $100.00 (Canadian students/residents). Foreign air speed delivery is included in all *Clinics* subscription prices. All prices are subject to change without notice. **POSTMASTER:** Send address changes to *Hand Clinics*, Elsevier Health Sciences Division, Subscription Customer Service, 3251 Riverport Lane, Maryland Heights, MO 63043. Customer Service (orders, claims, online, change of address): Elsevier Health Sciences Division, Subscription **Customer Service, 3251 Riverport Lane, Maryland Heights, MO 63043. Tel: 1-800-654-2452 (U.S. and Canada); 314-447-8871 (outside U.S. and Canada). Fax: 314-447-8029. E-mail: journalscustomerservice-usa@elsevier.com (for print support); journalsonlinesupport-usa@elsevier.com (for online support).**

Reprints. For copies of 100 or more of articles in this publication, please contact the Commercial Reprints Department, Elsevier Inc., 360 Park Avenue South, New York, New York 10010-1710. Tel.: 212-633-3874; Fax: 212-633-3820; E-mail: reprints@elsevier.com.

Hand Clinics is covered in *MEDLINE/PubMed (Index Medicus), Current Contents/Clinical Medicine, EMBASE/Excerpta Medica,* and *ISI/BIOMED.*

Contributors

CONSULTING EDITOR

KEVIN C. CHUNG, MD, MS
Charles B.G. de Nancrede Professor of Surgery, Professor of Plastic Surgery and Orthopaedic Surgery, Chief of Hand Surgery, Department of Surgery, Section of Plastic Surgery, Michigan Medicine, Assistant Dean for Faculty Affairs, Associate Director of Global REACH, University of Michigan Medical School, University of Michigan, The University of Michigan Health System, Ann Arbor, Michigan, USA

EDITORS

JIN BO TANG, MD
Professor and Chair, Department of Hand Surgery, The Hand Surgery Research Center, Affiliated Hospital of Nantong University, Nantong, Jiangsu, China

GREY GIDDINS, BA, MBBCh, FRCS (Orth)
Consultant Orthopaedic and Hand Surgeon, The Hand to Elbow Clinic, Royal United Hospital, Visiting Professor, University of Bath, Bath, United Kingdom; Editor-in-Chief, *Journal of Hand Surgery* (European) (2012–2016), Hunterian Professor 2021

AUTHORS

MICHEL E.H. BOECKSTYNS, MD, PhD
Senior Consultant, Hand Surgery, Capio PH, Hellerup, Denmark

COLTON BOUDREAU, MD
Division of Plastic Surgery, Dalhousie University, Halifax, Nova Scotia, Canada

KEVIN C. CHUNG, MD, MS
Charles B.G. de Nancrede Professor of Surgery, Professor of Plastic Surgery and Orthopaedic Surgery, Chief of Hand Surgery, Department of Surgery, Section of Plastic Surgery, Michigan Medicine, Assistant Dean for Faculty Affairs, Associate Director of Global REACH, University of Michigan Medical School, University of Michigan, The University of Michigan Health System, Ann Arbor, Michigan, USA

GREY GIDDINS, BA, MBBCh, FRCS (Orth)
Consultant Orthopaedic and Hand Surgeon, The Hand to Elbow Clinic, Royal United Hospital, Visiting Professor, University of Bath, Bath, United Kingdom

IGOR GOLUBEV, MD
National Medical Research Center of Traumatology and Orthopedics Named After N.N. Priorov, Moscow, Russia

DONALD LALONDE, MD, FRCSC
Professor, Surgery, Division of Plastic Surgery, Dalhousie University, Saint John, New Brunswick, Canada

ULRICH MENNEN, MBChB(Pret), FRCS(Glasg), FRCS(Edin), FCS(SA)Orth, MMed(Orth), FHMVS(DUMC), MD(Orth), DSc(Med)
Emeritus Professor of Hand Surgery, University of Pretoria and Jacaranda Hospital, Pretoria, South Africa; Editor, *IFFSH* Ezine

BRIAN W. STARR, MD
Hand Surgery Fellow, Section of Plastic Surgery, The University of Michigan Health System, Ann Arbor, Michigan, USA

JIN BO TANG, MD
Professor and Chair, Department of
Hand Surgery, The Hand Surgery
Research Center, Affiliated Hospital of
Nantong University, Nantong, Jiangsu,
China

EDUARDO R. ZANCOLLI III, MD
Professor in Hand Surgery, Argentine
Association for Hand Surgery
Specialists' Career, Buenos Aires,
Argentina

Contents

> Mallet injuries, either tendinous or bony, are common. They are often studied together and typically treated in the same way with extension splintage for 6 to 8 weeks. Yet the evidence clearly shows there are different injuries that present in the same way. Tendinous mallet injuries present in older patients usually following a low energy injury; they are often painless. The commonly injured fingers are the middle and ring. The injuries are almost always single digit without concomitant injuries. There is an extensor lag of a mean of 31^0 (range $3°–59^0$) in the patients treated in my unit. In contrast, bony mallet injuries occur at a younger age (mean 40 years) and are always due to high energy injuries. The injuries are always painful. The commonly injured fingers are the ring and little fingers. There are multiple injuries in 3% (range 2%–5%) and in 4% to 8% of cases, there are concomitant (nondigital) injuries according to data in my unit. Radiologically there is an appreciably smaller extensor lag; mean 13^0 (range $0°–40^0$). In particular, bony mallet injuries are extension compression, not avulsion, fractures which should not logically be treated with an extension splint which will reproduce the direction of injury.

> In recent decades, there has been a trend toward increased use of operative treatment of hand fractures. However, internal stabilization with wires or open reduction and internal fixation of the phalanges and the metacarpals carries a risk of surgical complications that can be avoided by using appropriate conservative treatment. In this article, some hand fractures that can be managed safely without surgery are discussed. In conclusion, when facing a fracture in the hand, the first consideration is whether the fracture can be treated nonoperatively and not which operative treatment is most appropriate. This applies to both displaced and undisplaced fractures.

> Field sterility for K-wire insertion outside the main operating room is much cheaper and greener (ie, there is less waste). It permits increased access to more affordable surgery because unnecessary sedation and full sterility are eliminated. Early pain-guided

protected movement of K-wired finger fractures at 3 to 5 days leads to less stiffness. It will not result in loss of reduction or infection around K-wires if patients avoid "pain" (ie, do not perform movements that hurt). Early protected movement and early removal of K-wires at 2 to 4 weeks contribute to less stiffness after operative hand/finger fracture reduction and stabilization.

It has long been thought that the surgical treatment of osteoarthritis of the first carpometacarpal joint must replicate the normal anatomy. Common sense argues that biomechanical stability can be achieved by a simple ball-and-socket joint obviating complicated ligament reconstructions and trapezium replacements. Our argument is presented and the conclusions are based on the results of a very large series over a long period. A simple trapezium excision arthroplasty of the base of the thumb without ligamentous reconstructions is all that needs to be done to surgically solve painful osteoarthritis of the first carpometacarpal joint. Anything more is overoperating.

 Video content accompanies this article at http://www.hand.theclinics.com.

The theoretic disadvantage of dynamic tendon transfers is the perception that they are "more complex" than static procedures. The latter may provide a simple solution to claw deformity in a subset of patients; however, they completely disregard the disability associated with loss of the intrinsic musculature. Dynamic procedures reconstruct in part the deficient intrinsic forces and are thus capable of correcting the deformity and some disabilities associated with ulnar nerve palsy. In our practice, we have consistently achieved reasonable correction of claw deformity and improvement in tendon synchrony and grip strength with a modified Stiles-Bunnell, flexor digitorum superficialis tendon transfer.

This article discusses ulnar, median, and radial nerve compression in the proximal forearm and elbow and some possible common misconceptions. In particular, the ligament of Struthers' extremely rarely causes ulnar neuropathy. Lacertus syndrome and flexor superficialis-pronator syndrome can be diagnosed separately. Surgical release can be through a small incision. Acronyms for compression to radial nerve in proximal forearm can be simplified to radial tunnel syndrome, which includes a mild type (classical radial tunnel syndrome) and a severe type (posterior interosseous nerve (PIN) compression).

Although patients with obstetric brachial plexus injuries (OBPI) have been recognized and treated for greater than 100 years there is much that is not understood or is mis-understood. I address 6 areas for discussion: the cause of OBPI and whether it matters to nerve surgeons; the value of the Narakas grading; whether surgeons should perform primary nerve surgery, especially in patients with incomplete OBPI; the cause and treatment of shoulder tightness; the cause and treatment of elbow contracture; and whether patients with OBPI need surgery in adulthood.

Direct Repair of Flexor Tendons Close to Bony Insertion and Ruptured Collateral Ligaments

337

Jin Bo Tang

Lacerated flexor tendons close to bony junction are commonly repaired using a pull-out suture. However, these injuries very close to the tendon-bone junction can be repaired with robust direct suture repair of the proximal tendon stump with the short residual tendon stump and any local tissues such as periosteum and joint volar plate. Subacute or chronic traumatic rupture at the midpart of the collateral ligaments can also be repaired by "refreshing" the divided ligament ends and repairing the ligament stumps to local tissues with multiple sutures often combined with tightening the elongated joint capsule.

Our Disagreement on "Iceberg View" on the Ulnar Wrist and Clinical Implications

343

Eduardo R. Zancolli III

The diagnosis of ulnar-sided wrist symptoms concentrates on distal radioulnar joint and triquetral-hamate joint pathology. I consider this is only looking at the "tip of the iceberg" and ignoring other possible pathologies. In particular, this ignores the role of triquetrohamate and pisotriquetral pathologies. I outline our approaches to these pathologies noting the important ligamentous structures, the clinical presentations, the relevant investigations, and the surgical treatments and outcomes that I have found to be reliable. I would encourage hand surgeons to think more widely about ulnar-sided wrist symptoms, in particular triquetrohamate and pisotriquetral joint instabilities.

Slight Elongation of the Scaphoid and Cancellous Bone Graft Without Compression for Treatment of Scaphoid Nonunions

351

Igor Golubev

In treating scaphoid nonunion, we have developed a technique of bone grafting and elongation of the scaphoid stabilizing the construct with K wires without compression. Bony union was achieved in the large majority of scaphoids as demonstrated on computed tomography (CT) scans. We advocate slight lengthening of the scaphoid with bone graft and K-wire fixation without compression of the grafted bone when treating scaphoid waist nonunion.

10 Hypotheses in Hand Surgery

357

Jin Bo Tang

I have put together 10 topics and labeled them as hypotheses, which outline my preferred practices. The topics relate to questionable nerve compression, double crush syndrome of nerves, motion therapy after surgery, delayed primary tendon repair, proximal pole fracture of the scaphoid, short splint, and indications for postoperative hand elevation. I found no proof whether my preferred methods are better than or inferior to alternative methods that others use. The 10 hypotheses are presented to stimulate thinking, clinical observation, or investigations and highlight several areas of research. Investigation into these hypotheses may avoid unnecessary treatment or improve postsurgical comfort for patients and long-term outcomes of treatment.

HAND CLINICS

SERIES OF RELATED INTEREST:

Clinics in Plastic Surgery
https://www.plasticsurgery.theclinics.com/

Orthopedic Clinics of North America
https://www.orthopedic.theclinics.com/

Clinics in Sports Medicine
http://www.sportsmed.theclinics.com/

THE CLINICS ARE AVAILABLE ONLINE!
Access your subscription at:
www.theclinics.com

Preface
Challenge the Current Wisdom of Hand Surgery

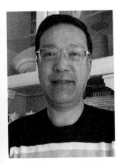

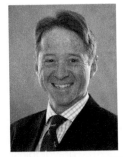

Jin Bo Tang, MD   Grey Giddins, BA, MBBCh, FRCS (Orth)
Editors

As clinicians and humans, we both favor tradition and embrace novelty, although not all to the same degree. We believe the "established" facts taught to us by our trainers, but also readily take on new treatments where we think they will improve the outcomes for our patients. Sometimes these "established" facts or new treatments are less proven than we realize yet we may struggle to resist their siren calls; undoubtedly there is an emotional as well as an intellectual content to our practices.

One of the most striking of these traditional beliefs, which has now been disproven, is the advice not to use adrenaline for peripheral local anesthetic injections. Don Lalonde has led this work and provides further evidence in this issue of the opportunities available for treating patients under local anesthetic and questions further beliefs, particularly the need to undertake K-wiring procedures in a main operating theater, fully gowned. Other beliefs are also challenged in this issue.

It is clearly shown that bony and tendinous mallet injuries are different injuries presenting in the same way, with an extensor lag, and should not be treated the same or reported together in scientific studies. Ulrich Mennen challenges the belief that we should now move on from trapeziectomy as a treatment for thumb-base arthritis and instead look to the various arthroplasties that are now available. Based upon his considerable experience, he feels that the main trapeziectomy is simple, reliable, and inexpensive and should not be rejected in favor of novelty. Michel Boeksteyns highlights how effective nonoperative treatment can be for most hand fractures. Undoubtedly the way to turn a fracture into a disaster most reliably is to operate. This does not mean there is no role for surgery, but surgeons need to be aware of what can be achieved nonoperatively and measure their practice against that to ensure that their patients are doing appreciably better to justify surgical intervention. This raises the philosophical question of how many patients need to be a little better from surgery to make up for the occasional patient who is substantially worse?

The articles are not just about challenging new practices; rather they also introduce new ideas challenging older ways of practicing. There is increasing interest in minimal access surgery for less common nerve entrapment potentially reducing the complications but requiring precise preoperative assessment to define the site of nerve entrapment. Edouard Zancolli introduces some new ideas on ulnar-sided wrist pathology outside the conventional thinking of the distal radioulnar joint, the triangular fibrocartilaginous complex, pisotriquetral joint arthritis, and extensor carpi ulnaris tendinopathy. Obstetric brachial plexus injuries are uncommon but potentially devastating. There is considerable variation in practice and beliefs among surgeons who treat these patients not least about the causes of shoulder joint tightness and its treatment and the likelihood of patients requiring further surgery in later adulthood; some of these beliefs are challenged based upon established and new data.

We hope you enjoy reading these challenging ideas. You will not necessarily accept all of them,

Hand Clin 38 (2022) ix–x
https://doi.org/10.1016/j.hcl.2022.04.004
0749-0712/22/© 2022 Published by Elsevier Inc.

but do try to keep an open mind, as the authors have all thought hard about their practices and are trying to improve them for the benefit of their patients. We would encourage you to keep challenging your own practices and especially your long-held beliefs, which may not be proven, but at the same time look with some skepticism at new practices, which may not remain current throughout your career.

A unique feature of this collection is that all but two of the articles are authored by only one author, who is very senior and has decades of experience in the topic he discusses. The other two articles also reflect the practice of the senior authors. These authors and their preferred practices and rationales merit deliberate consideration. We are greatly indebted to them for their invaluable work on the articles in this issue, which represent a distillation of some of their career-long practice and thoughts.

Jin Bo Tang, MD
Department of Hand Surgery
The Hand Surgery Research Center
Affiliated Hospital of Nantong University
20 West Temple Road
Nantong 226001, Jiangsu, China

Grey Giddins, BA, MBBCh, FRCS (Orth)
The Hand to Elbow Clinic
29a James Street West
Bath BA1 2BT, UK

E-mail addresses:
jinbotang@yahoo.com (J.B. Tang)
greygiddins@handtoelbow.com (G. Giddins)

Editorial

Evidence-Based, Eminence-Based, Hypothesis-Based, or Wrong Information–Based Practice?

Healthcare givers—including those in hand surgery—are commonly considered to deliver their clinical treatment to patients based on evidence, eminence, or a combination of both, in order to obtain the best possible diagnoses and treatments. Therefore, correct clinical practice is often described as evidence- or eminence-based practice. I consider that two other categories of clinical practice exist but have not drawn sufficient attention. They are *hypothesis-based practice* and *wrong information–based practice*.

Hypothesis-based practice, using surgery as an example, is seen in two situations. The first is when treating rare and relatively uncommon disorders. The caregivers have no evidence or no reliable evidence to base treatment, even in consultation with senior colleagues, who also have neither evidence nor experience to support the practice they will give. They have to decide a treatment based on rationales or guesses and hypothesize that their treatment is the best according to the doctor's understanding, knowledge, and reasoning. The expertise level of even senior caregivers on these particular clinical problems can only be level II according to classification of Tang and Giddins.[1] There are no experts or experienced specialists. The second situation is when the treatment method is new and therefore experimental without evidence or eminence to support.

Wrong information–based practice exists more commonly than we recognize. The caregivers decide to use a clinical treatment based on published clinical data or conclusions, which are wrong in reality. The most detrimental are published false or largely unreliable clinical data and outcomes. Caregivers have no way to know that the information is false. These false reports are ideally caught before publication or retracted after the problems are exposed. In reality, detection of such problems is difficult, and sometimes even with solid facts of major misconducts of the authors, some journals do not act to retract or correct the published papers. This problem is worsened by emergence of a large number of journals of low quality or predatory in nature, which publish articles after loose peer-review and lenient editorial processes. Some of these journals are included in search engines, which makes suspicious data weigh similarly with those published in authoritative or serious journals. This is an emerging serious issue in the recent decade with expansion of literature, because not many colleagues look into or realize stringency of different journals.

Systematic reviews are often subject to journal stringency. The criteria for inclusion or exclusion of articles under systematic review do not include whether a journal is authoritative or predatory. A systematic review is itself a secondary analysis of original data with an inherent weakness: errors in interpretation of the original data are doubled. This weakness copied with uncertainties in selection criteria often makes such reviews too weak. I would trust and rely on those reports of trusted journals and trusted author teams more than on systematic reviews on the same topics. There appears to be a need to revise criteria for systematic reviews.

The above concerns might not be problems in the early 1990s when evidence-based medicine was advocated by Eddy.[2] With increases in the sources of evidence, issues of seriously analyzing the sources are critical. General practitioners often rely on "evidence" in the reports but have little insight to the information sources. Even caregivers in an academic institute may not be able to discern or easily suspect false information because of general trust on academic journals and the belief that they are strict.

As journals grow in number markedly, I see two other types of journals positioned between what are called authoritative (serious) journals and predatory journals. One includes those with excellent peer reviews and editorial process, but they lack rigorous measures to minimize publication of wrong information. Another are journals bearing some features of the predatory ones and which are run by less-trained editors; these journals have little or no capability of preventing, correcting, or retracting misinformation. I consider above

Hand Clin 38 (2022) xi–xii
https://doi.org/10.1016/j.hcl.2022.04.005
0749-0712/22/© 2022 Published by Elsevier Inc.

4 groups or types of journals of varying stringency exist. These 4 types may be called *serious, dependable, lenient*, or *predatory* journals, respectively. The latter two may have a high risk of misinformation.

Besides, clinical outcome reports may make improper or imprecise final conclusions based on correct data and correct study process. The problems often lie in the interpretation of findings and data and the wordings used. Whether these improper or imprecise conclusions are finally published depends on the quality of the editorial review process. In my experience as an editor, I have to raise questions to the authors for the wordings of conclusions or revise them myself after rounds of peer review and revisions. Sometimes the authors are ones who are quite senior, frequently published, or both. I can see that if I had not questioned or revised these conclusions, errors would be published and affect the selection of clinical methods by the readers. Clinical evidence in these reports is valid, but the interpretation of the evidence is imprecise or improper.

The best way to decrease wrong information relating to data interpretation in a report is to place much attention on checking the final conclusions. This is important because most readers would only read the conclusions, not sensibly check whether the data actually led to the conclusions. Therefore, before publication, the scope of the conclusions should be carefully scaled without overgeneralization, and limitations should be clearly presented before making any final conclusions. If expert peer-reviewers and editors fail to revise the conclusions, general readers are unlikely to do so. I have encountered several occasions in which I found that the data led to almost entirely opposite conclusions from those made by the authors. I wrote so to the authors, and they changed the conclusions.

To clearly recognize the imperfect sites where wrong information may be introduced would cause providers to be more careful in adopting "evidence" reported. Among "evidence" they read and use, some may be false at the data collection and reporting levels at the worst, which may be a small part of the literature. Some are from reliable and correct studies, but misinterpretation causes problems. Recognition would highlight the potential problems in the literature and alert the readers.

Recognition of these problems does not undermine the importance of the medical literature and the collective efforts of all involved. Rather it raises awareness of the need to clean the literature overall and to provide *correct interpretation and conclusions* in individual reports, a task of authors, reviewers, editors, and postpublication commenting. This is essential to preventing wrong information. Once a wrong conclusion is printed, it is hard to change, which is often cited to argue against the authentic evidence and weaken its impact on clinical decision making. The peer review and editorial process are not perfect and will never be. It is best to let junior colleagues know very clearly about the process' fallibility. Once printed, these articles carry a degree of authority, especially to the junior caregivers. It is often easier to critique a paper with senior academic practitioners because they examine and have insight themselves. Junior ones rely more heavily on what is printed, and consequently, the impact on them is not easily changed.

In summary, I bring hypothesis-based practice and wrong information-based practice to wide attention, and I group journals by 4 different levels of stringency. I urge colleagues to recognize these when seeking or applying evidence in delivering patient care.

Jin Bo Tang, MD
Department of Hand Surgery
Affiliated Hospital of Nantong University
20 West Temple Road
Nantong 226001, Jiangsu, China

E-mail address:
jinbotang@yahoo.com

REFERENCES

1. Tang JB, Giddins G. Why and how to report surgeons' levels of expertise. J Hand Surg Eur 2016;41:365–6.
2. Eddy DM. A manual for assessing health practices and designing practice policies. West Philadelphia, PA: American College of Physicians; 1992.

Editorial
"Established" Rules or Teachings Are Less Proven than We Realize

Professor Grey Giddins wrote most of the preface of this book. I only added a few more lines in its final paragraph. I am very touched by what Professor Grey Giddins wrote, especially the lines that I quote below. I believe this deserves attention from all our colleagues.

'We believe the "established" facts taught to us by our trainers, but also readily take on new treatments where we think they will improve the outcomes for our patients. Sometimes these "established" facts or new treatments are less proven than we realize.' — Grey Giddins

I expand on these lines with a few examples below; these exemplify how our readers may need to examine their practices from time to time and assess the teachings or routines on which their practices are based. Many therapists and hand surgeons use "10 runs of active flexion exercises in each exercise session" and instruct patients to perform hourly motion exercise after flexor tendon repair. This exercise regimen and frequencies are deeply rooted in therapists' minds and in protocols of many therapy units. Where did the "10 runs" come from? Are the "10 runs" supported by evidence? I recall the "10 runs" stemmed from a paper in 1989, one of the earliest reports of active flexion motion after zone 2 flexor tendon repair, where "two passive and four active movements was repeated every four hours during the day."[1] Was there any evidence in the report of 1989 to support why the authors used 6 runs at that time? No, it was just what the authors did for their patients. The authors could have used 20 or 30 runs at that time instead. I do not know why they used only 6 runs per session. I presume the authors considered early active flexion was a new idea, so fewer runs were safer; 6 was rounded to 10 later.

The 10 runs and hourly motion have dominated the early active motion protocols for the next 30 years in many units; they have been written up widely especially in major textbooks. The importance of increasing the number of runs beyond 10 runs to many more runs (>30 or 40) in each session were later recognized in order to make therapy efficient.[2-4] I found it took surgeons from different institutes considerable effort to make

their local therapists or surgeons update the protocol to 30 or 40 runs, instead of 10 runs, because they had been brought up with the teachings of 10 runs, which seems only based on a random decision decades ago. For many people, change is difficult after being taught, especially by respected trainers or recognized authorities on a subject. The hypothetic *better treatments* are often no better than guesses.

There are many other examples. The reported indications for the operative correction of angulation at second to fifth metacarpal necks vary from 20° to 50°. Is the recommendation of 40° of angulation for the fourth metacarpal neck supported by any evidence? No, it is a suggestion or a guess. For any metacarpal neck fracture, if hand function is good, the angulation is not a major consideration for offering surgery. Palmar inclination (dorsal angulation) of the metacarpal neck often does not interfere with hand function, as there is a natural palmar inclination from the metacarpal base to the fingertip that favors hand grip. Another example is internal fixation of scaphoid; compression of the two fractured parts is commonly recommended. However, especially with bone grafting, fixing the scaphoid fracture *without compression* may be equally good, or perhaps improve the healing rate, because little or no compression may favor local nutrition and perfusion. The current teachings of compression in fixating scaphoid fracture may be partly or entirely wrong.

Recently, a colleague talked about his mentor on his fellowship 15 years ago and commented that his mentor did many things differently from traditional teachings usually with improved outcomes. He considered the better outcomes were from this mentor's technical expertise and surgical judgment as well as unique insights into the disorders he treats beyond what is written in the textbooks. Often the chapter authors of textbooks are less experienced or learned than this very senior surgeon. The textbooks almost imply that if a very senior (expert) hand surgeon does many standard procedures, his or her outcomes would be no better than those obtained by a hand surgeon just finishing fellowship. Yet years or

Hand Clin 38 (2022) xiii–xiv
https://doi.org/10.1016/j.hcl.2022.04.006
0749-0712/22/© 2022 Published by Elsevier Inc.

decades of practice should lead to another level of expertise, and more personalized approaches are developed. Clearly, master surgeons are more or less unique in their clinical or surgical methods.

Our colleagues should really keep an open mind and realize that many "firm" practices are often those earlier colleagues *chose to do*. The textbook authors describe what they have read or were taught and add their own new suggestions. They may fail to clearly label them with "… is a suggestion without strong support of good evidence" or "the current major practice is ….. , but these are only recommendations and not fully proven." Often what is written in textbooks is a presentation of personal methods *without any stipulation of degree of certainty*.

I urge colleagues to find more examples and challenge them! This does not mean we have no respect for the current rules or methods, or no respect for the textbooks, which carry important messages based on the collective work of many authorities, but the contents cannot be entirely proven and may not be correct. Keeping an open mind and seeking to understand where the recommended treatments come from would further improve clinical practice beyond what one learns from books. With a similar approach, you can contribute to validate these current methods or modify them through your studies.

Though the textbook authors do not commonly stipulate given "rules," whether they are suggestions based on limited factual information, thoughts, or proven facts, these books are often the basis for forming examination questions for a range of qualifications. The designed answers are often changed or radicalized with soft recommendations transformed into seemingly undisputable rules in the form of answers. For the colleagues who are open to learning, they may understand the limitations of examination questions, and some would use these as a starting point to change the practices and challenging the dogma. Unfortunately, many others consider these answers as "rules" and stick to them rigidly; others may stick firmly to what they learn early in their training even when they are more senior. Actually these answers in qualification examination only serve as rough guidelines to those who have little experience to judge or design their independent treatment strategies. The qualification examination only ensures no major mistakes will be committed by the young practitioners, but these are often distanced from the best clinical treatments, especially the carefully designed personalized treatment plan and decision making of an experienced practitioner based on more updated frontier knowledge and own experience.

I suggest a statement be added at the beginning of qualification examinations, such as: *The correct answers are based on mainstream recommendations in the country or continent where the test is taken. Some correct answers may lack strong support with evidence or are not proven adequately.* This statement would reflect the nature of test questions and answers and act as a reminder to examiners and examinees to test the answers as rigorously as possible in their own practices. I see many young colleagues do not realize the limitations and nature of these tests. If there was a chance to offer advice as a gift to graduating trainees, this would be it.

In the real world, the level of certainty in clinical recommendation is often insufficiently understood, and dogma dominates the practice of even experienced colleagues. There is a lack of awareness of the weak evidential support of many current practices. However, it is through challenging and changing these seemingly "correct rules" that our profession will advance. The later generation of hand surgeons will readily understand the errors in our current methods and wonder why these were not understood or revised by the previous generation of hand surgeons that is, our generation, similar to how we now think about the practices and people who worked 20 or 30 years ahead of us in this specialty.

Jin Bo Tang, MD
Department of Hand Surgery
Affiliated Hospital of Nantong University
20 West Temple Road
Nantong 226001, Jiangsu, China

E-mail address:
jinbotang@yahoo.com

REFERENCES

1. Cullen KW, Tolhurst P, Lang D, et al. Flexor tendon repair in zone 2 followed by controlled active mobilisation. J Hand Surg Br 1989;14:392–5.
2. Tang JB. Indications, methods, postoperative motion and outcome evaluation of primary flexor tendon repairs in zone 2. J Hand Surg Eur 2007;32:118–29.
3. Tang JB, Zhou X, Pan ZJ, et al. Strong digital flexor tendon repair, extension-flexion test, and early active flexion: experience in 300 tendons. Hand Clin 2017;33:455–63.
4. Tang JB. Rehabilitation after flexor tendon repair and others: a safe and efficient protocol. J Hand Surg Eur 2021;46:813–7.

Mallet Finger
Two Different Injuries

Grey Giddins, MBBCh, FRCS (Orth)[a,b,c,*]

KEYWORDS

• Mallet • Tendinous • Bony • Mechanism of injury • Subluxation

KEY POINTS

- Mallet injuries, either tendinous or bony, are common. They are often studied together and typically treated in the same way with extension splintage for 6-8 weeks. Yet the evidence clearly shows there are different injuries which present in the same way.
- Tendinous mallet injuries present in older patients usually following a low energy injury; they are often painless.
- The injuries are almost always affect a single digit without concomitant injuries.
- Bony mallet injuries occur at a younger age (mean 40 years) and are always due high energy injuries. The injuries are always painful.
- There are multiple injuries in 3 (range 2-5)% and in 4-8% of cases there are concomitant (non-digital) injuries according to data in my unit.
- In particular bony mallet injuries are extension compression, not avulsion, fractures which should not logically be treated with an extensor splint which will reproduce the direction of injury.
- Reseearch studies should not conflate these injuries or they are likely to be invalid

INTRODUCTION

Mallet finger is a common injury presenting with an extensor lag at the distal inter-phalangeal (DIP) joint. The 2 main causes are tendinous, that is, a rupture or division of the extensor tendon (typically a closed injury) or bony (**Fig. 1**). The former is assumed to be caused by loading the DIP joint while it is being flexed; the latter is typically referred to as an avulsion injury implying the same mechanism. On this basis these are biomechanically the same injury and so warrant the same treatment, that is, extension/hyper-extension splintage until extensor integrity is restored.

Some authors have previously suggested that bony mallet Injuries are impaction fractures.[1,2] The mechanism would be a hyper-extension rather than a hyper-flexion injury. Hyper-extension splintage, for example, with a Stack splint (**Fig. 2**) would, therefore, be illogical as it would risk exacerbating the original injury. In addition any studies considering these injuries would risk drawing incorrect conclusions as they would be treating different injuries; this would be like treating Colles' type (extension) distal radius fractures and Smith's type (flexion) distal radius fractures in the same ways which would be considered inappropriate.

The aim of this article is to consider the evidence that these are different injuries and so warrant different treatments and to raise questions about their cause and treatment. I will consider the mechanisms of injury, the radiographic presentations, and previous studies.

MECHANISMS OF INJURY

A prospective study was performed of patients with tendinous and bony mallet injuries[3] assessing their mechanisms of injury. These were categorized into low or high-energy injuries. In doubt, the injuries were classified as high energy for

[a] The Hand to Elbow Clinic, Bath, Bath, United Kingdom; [b] Royal United Hospital, Bath, United Kingdom;
[c] University of Bath, Bath, United Kingdom
* University of Bath, Bath, United Kingdom.
E-mail address: greygiddins@handtoelbow.com

Hand Clin 38 (2022) 281–288
https://doi.org/10.1016/j.hcl.2022.02.005
0749-0712/22/© 2022 Elsevier Inc. All rights reserved.

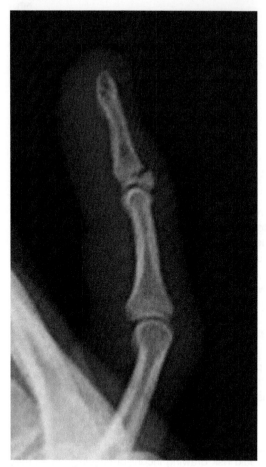

Fig. 1. Lateral radiograph showing a bony mallet injury.

tendinous mallet injuries and low-energy for bony mallet injuries to minimize bias. Low energy mechanisms of injury descriptions included putting on socks or changing bed linen; high energy injury descriptions included missed catches and falls. Of note 19% of patients with tendinous mallet injuries reported no pain at the time of injury, they just became aware of an extensor lag.[3] Outcomes were not reviewed as that was not the purpose of the study.

Sixty-two patients presented with tendinous mallet injuries and 83 patients with bony mallet injuries in patients treated in my unit in recent years. Of the patients with tendinous injuries, only 12 of

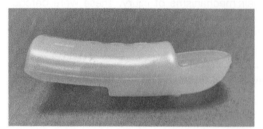

Fig. 2. Stack splint.

62 (18%) suffered possible high energy injuries; the remaining 50 (82%) suffered low-energy injuries and 12 (19%) noted no pain. The patients with bony mallet injuries all had high-energy injuries. Two patients suffered bony mallet injuries in 2 fingers and 7 patients (8%) had other concomitant fractures. The incidence of multiple bony mallet injuries in my unit is comparable with the series of Moradi and colleagues[4] who reported multiple mallet injuries in 9 of 383 (2%) patients, Weber and Schneider[5] who reported 2 double injuries in 42 patients (5%) and Trickett and colleagues[6] who reported multiple fractures in 7 of 211 (3%) digits (including 113 thumbs). Overall where reported in the literature multiple bony mallet injuries occurred in 20 of 719 patients, that is, 3% (range 2%–5%).

These data show that tendinous mallet injuries are predominantly low energy injuries as has been shown by almost all other published series, except Facca and colleagues,[7] (**Table 1**) while bony mallet injuries are all high-energy injuries as also shown by Botero and colleagues.[8] Patients with tendinous mallet injuries are a mean of 17 years older than patients with bony mallet injuries. This has been suggested previously by Moss and Steingold,[9,10] but never shown so clearly. Men were more often injured in both groups reported as published previously[3] (see **Table 1**). Tendinous mallet injuries affected predominantly the middle and ring fingers while bony mallet injuries affected predominantly the ring and little fingers as also shown in other studies (see **Table 1**).

In this series, there were 7 (8%) appreciable concomitant injuries in the bone mallet group further highlighting the higher energy nature of bony mallet injuries and the risk of overlooking concomitant injuries. This association had not previously been reported, but has been confirmed in the study of Trickett and colleagues[6] who reported 8 (4%) patients with polytrauma in their series of 211 patients with bony mallet injuries. In no patients with low-energy injuries was there a substantial fracture fragment as opposed to a minor avulsion fracture. Therefore, in patients with a clear history of low energy injury and a mallet deformity, radiographs seem to be unnecessary.

RADIOLOGICAL ASSESSMENT

I have also measured the extensor lag of the DIP joint in the acute (postinjury) radiographs following bony and tendinous mallet injuries in patients presenting to our hospital and the sizes of the bony fragments in the patients with bony mallet injuries using the electronic Picture Archiving and

Table 1
Published data re. bony and tendinous mallet injuries

Authors	No of Injuries	Mean Age (Range) in Years	Gender M = Male F = Female	Right (R)/ Left (L)	Index	Middle	Ring	Little	Fragment Size Mean (Range) %	Mechanism		
										Sport	Other high energy (or not defined)	Low energy or unknown
Bony mallet injuries												
Weber and Schneider,[5] 1983[a]	43	42 (5–61)	M31:F10		3	16	12	10	48 (15–100)	21	23	0
Damron and Engber,[21] 1983	19	23(17–32)	M13:F6						51 (38–67)	16	3	0
Pegoli et al,[29–31] 2004	65	28 (12–71)		40/25	20	20	15	10		42	23	0
Darder-Prats et al,[22–28] 1998	22	23 (14–34)	M18:F4						4 < 1/3	All falls or sports		0
Facca et al,[7] 2007[b]	115 (fingers with c 2 thumbs)			61% = R70:L45	11% = 13	26% = 30	28% = 33	35.4% = 41				
Moradi et al,[4] 2016	383	43 (SD 16)	M225:F167	209/183	45	77	134	136	46 (SD14)		76%	24%
Trickett et al,[6] 2021	218 digits; 205 fingers (211 patients)	NR	M131: F80	NR	14	35	72	84				

(continued on next page)

Table 1
(continued)

Authors	No of Injuries	Mean Age (Range) in Years	Gender M = Male F = Female	Right (R)/ Left (L)	Index	Middle	Ring	Little	Fragment Size Mean (Range) %	Mechanism
This article	85	40(12–70)	M46:F37	48/37	8	16	26	35	51 (range 29–83) 21	64 0
Total for bony injuries (%)	732	33	M 464:F 304 (60:40)	398/301 (57:43)	103 (11%)	195 (22%)	292(32%)	316(35%)		
Tendinous injuries										
Facca et al,[7] 2007[b]	144 (fingers with c 9 thumbs)	1.26 that is,. M80:F64	54% = R78:L66	4% = 6	38.7% = 59	30% = 45	22% = 34	61%	39%
Vernet et al,[7] 2019[c]	100	Age 47 (21–78)	60:40	R70:L29	4	35	40	20		
This article	62	Age 55 (14–90)	44:18	R39:L 23	2	31	20	9	12	50
Total for tendinous	306	50	184:122 (60:40)	R 187: L 118 (61:39)	12 (4%)	125 (41%)	105 (34%)	63 (21%)		

[a] This article only recorded the fingers of 41 injuries.
[b] The percentages of injured fingers were taken from graphs that were a little difficult to read so may be inaccurate by 1% to 2%. The exact % to one decimal point was taken from the text of the article.
[c] The article reported on 100 cases but one case is missing in the tables of cases.

Communications System (PACS). I measured the DIP joint extensor lag as the angle of the middle of the shaft of the distal phalanx relative to the long axis of the middle of the shaft of the middle phalanx (**Fig. 3**). Some original postinjury radiographs were not available and in some patients, their finger had been supported by support making measurement unreliable; I excluded these data. The size of the dorsal bony fracture fragments was measured and recorded as a percentage of the base of the distal phalanx on the lateral radiograph.[11]

I have reviewed 79 patients with 79 tendinous mallet injuries and 103 patients with 108 bony mallet injuries many of whom were included in the study on mechanisms of injury. I could measure 63 fingers in the 79 patients (79 fingers) with tendinous injuries; they had a mean radiological extensor lag of 31^0 (range 3°–59^0). Twelve patients had a small bony avulsion; these patients had a mean extensor lag of 34^0 (range 21°–57^0). I could

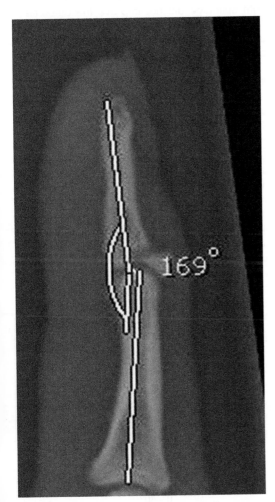

Fig. 3. Extensor lag measured on the PACS system.

measure 90 fingers in 103 patients (108 fingers) with bony mallet injuries; they had a mean extensor lag of 13^0 (range 0°–40^0) ($P < .001$). The mean sizes of the fracture fragments were 52 (range 24–80) %; in none was the fracture fragment less than 24% and in only 5 (5%) was the fracture fragment 1/3 (33%) or less. There was no correlation between fracture fragment size and measured extensor lag (**Fig. 4**).

DISCUSSION

Previously Hoch and colleagues[12] and Kreuder and colleagues[13] showed that it is unlikely that there would be avulsion of a large intra-articular fracture fragment by DIP joint hyperflexion. Hoch and colleagues[12] analyzed the microscopic anatomy of the extensor mechanism and concluded that the extent of the distal attachment of the extensor mechanism over the back of the distal phalanx and into the nail plate would make a complete failure of the extensor mechanism unlikely even in the presence of a large bony fracture fragment. This fits with the significantly less extensor lag in bony than tendinous mallet injuries. Kreuder and colleagues[13] undertook an in vitro study whereby they hit the end of 103 fresh human cadaver fingers with a weighted pendulum with the DIP joints in flexion or extension. Of the 49 flexion injuries 5 (10%) had rupture of the extensor mechanism and six (12%) had bony avulsions of the dorsal tip of the distal phalanx not involving the joint surface. Of the 54 fingers loaded in extension 2 (4%) had dorsal impaction fractures extending onto the joint surface as seen with bony mallet injuries. Five of the fingers loaded into flexion and extension were analyzed histologically. Of the extension loaded fingers one had no dorsal failure but the tearing of the palmar plate; this fits with the subluxation of the distal phalanx in some cases of bony mallet injuries which is associated with pivoting on lateral extension radiographs[11] which almost certainly requires failure of the palmar plate of the DIP joint.

The data show that there is significantly less DIP joint extensor lag with bony mallet injuries than tendinous mallet injuries further indicating that these are not avulsion injuries. Were bony mallet injuries avulsion injuries there should be similar or greater extensor lag than with tendinous mallet injuries, especially with large fragment injuries as there would be some collateral ligament damage. Avulsion injuries should logically pull off a range of fragment sizes typically smaller rather than larger bone fragments. Therefore, there should be a range of fragment sizes from 1% upwards with higher numbers at the lower percentages. Yet in the study,

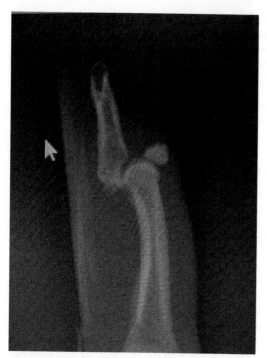

Fig. 4. Graph showing no correlation between fracture fragment size and extensor lag.

there were no fracture fragments smaller than 24%. The evidence that bony mallet injuries are impaction injuries is further challenged by the paper of Giddins and Giddins[14] describing the upper limb falling reflex; this showed that adults typically land first on their fingertips when they fall. When this sophisticated reflex fails some people will land on their extended fingertips helping to explain the frequency of finger injuries in general and of DIP joint impaction injuries in particular. Trickett and colleagues[6] reported that no patients specifically described a hyperflexion injury in their series but 9 clearly described a hyper-extension injury.

This information matters because misunderstanding mechanisms of injury may lead to inappropriate treatment: a bony mallet injury that occurs due to a hyperextension force should not logically be treated with a Stack splint which applies a hyperextension force (appropriate for a tendinous mallet injury) as this potentially increases the risk of subluxation of the distal phalanx[11] as previously suggested by McMinn[1] and Engber and Lange.[2] Furthermore, assuming this hypothesis is correct they are such dissimilar injuries (although presenting with an extensor lag) that they should not be classified together as in the Doyle[15] or Tubiana[16] classifications which merely confuse by merging these injuries. In addition any research studies conflating the 2 types of injuries such as historically Abouna and Brown[17] or Moss and Steingold[9] and more recently the randomized controlled study of Gruber at al.[18–20] risk drawing incorrect conclusions as they effectively treated 2 very different injuries. In particular, the study of Gruber and colleagues[18] showed that night splintage did not improve the outcome of these injuries. As they assessed both tendinous and bony mallet injuries together their conclusions must be in doubt.

Logically bony mallet injuries should be splinted straight or in slight flexion to reduce the risk of distal phalanx subluxation. This can be assessed with hyper-extension stress testing.[11] The author showed that with extension stress testing the main distal phalanx fragment glided or pivoted. If it glided there seems to be minimal risk of joint subluxation. If it pivoted there was a risk of joint subluxation. In these cases, surgical stabilization may be required although the recent study of Trickett and colleagues[6] would suggest not. The subluxation on extension stress testing also indicates these are hyper-extension impaction fractures as the pivoting must require some injury to

Table 2 Differences between tendinous and bony mallet injuries		
	Tendinous Injury	**Bony Injury**
Mean age (years)	57	40
Mechanism	Mainly low energy injury	"Always" high energy injury
Pain at injury	Often painless 19%	Always painful
Injured digits	Mainly middle and ring fingers	Mainly ring and little fingers
Concomitant injuries	Infrequent	4%–8% other fractures
Multiple digits	Rare	Mean 3 (range 2–5)%
Extensor lag on initial radiographs	Mean: 31° Range: 3°–59°	13° 0°–40°

the volar structures[13] which would not occur with an avulsion fracture.

Recent work in our hospital suggests that after 4 weeks the dorsal fracture fragment moves with the main fragment of the distal phalanx, that is, stability has been restored to the DIP joint. This suggests that extension splinting for bony mallet injuries need only last 4 weeks for some and perhaps all of these injuries which would fit with bone healing times in the hand. In contrast, the much slower extensor tendon healing time demands a longer period (6–8 weeks) of splintage for tendinous mallet injuries. The recent work of Trickett and colleagues treating 218 bony mallet injuries with splintage suggests they "never" need surgery.[6] That would fit with bony mallet injuries being more stable than tendinous mallet injuries as shown by the much lesser extensor lag but does not explain the outcome for the rarer but recognized cases of distal phalanx proximal volar dislocation (see **Fig. 4**). The differences between tendinous and bony mallet injuries are highlighted in **Table 2**.

SUMMARY

In summary, tendinous and bony mallet injuries are very different injuries presenting with the same clinical feature, that is, an extensor lag; this is highlighted in **Table 1**. Bony mallet injuries are hyperextension injuries so should not be treated with hyper-extension splints. Splints in neutral or slight flexion are theoretically preferable. They are probably only needed for 3 to 4 weeks allowing for earlier mobilization based on experience in the patients in my unit. In contrast, the much slower extensor tendon healing time demands a longer period (6–8 weeks) of splintage in extension for tendinous mallet injuries. Trickett and colleagues treated 218 bony mallet injuries with splintage and suggest they never need surgery. Research studies should not conflate these injuries or may be invalid.

REFERENCES

1. Lange RH, Engber WD. Hyperextension mallet finger. Orthopedics 1983;6:1426–31.
2. McMinn D. Mallet finger and fractures. Injury 1981; 12:477–9.
3. Giddins GE Tendinous and bony mallet finger: mechanisms of injury. J Hand Surg Eur 2021;46: 682–4.
4. Moradi A, Braun Y, Oflazoglu K, et al. Factors associated with subluxation in mallet fracture. J Hand Surg Eur 2017;42:176–81.
5. Wehbé MA, Schneider LH. Mallet fractures. J Bone Joint Surg Am 1984;66:658–69.
6. Trickett RW, Brock J, Shewring DJ. The non-operative management of bony mallet injuries. J Hand Surg Eur 2021;46:460–5.
7. Facca S, Nonnenmacher P, Liverneaux P. Treatment of mallet finger with dorsal nail glued splint: retrospective analysis of 270 cases. Rev Chir Orthop Reparatrice Appar Mot 2007;93:682–9.
8. Salazar Botero S, Hidalgo Diaz JJ, Benaïda A, et al. Review of acute traumatic closed mallet finger injuries in adults. Arch Plast Surg 2016;43:134–44.
9. Moss JG, Steingold RF. The long term results of mallet finger injury: a retrospective study of one hundred cases. Hand 1983;15:151–4.
10. Giddins GE. Radiographic comparison of bony and tendinous mallet injuries. J Hand Surg Eur 2022;47: 321–2.
11. Giddins GE. Bony mallet finger injuries: assessment of stability with extension stress testing. J Hand Surg Eur 2016;41:696–700.
12. Hoch J, Fritsch H, Frenz C. Does osseous extensor tendon avulsion or rupture really exist? Histologic plastination studies of insertion of the extensor aponeurosis and significance for operative therapy. Chirurg 1999;70:705–12.
13. Kreuder A, Pennig D, Boese CK, et al. Mallet finger: a simulation and analysis of hyperflexion versus hyperextension injuries. Surg Radiol Anat 2016;38: 403–7.
14. Giddins GE, Giddins H. Wrist and hand postures when falling and description of the upper limb falling reflex. Injury 2021;52:869–76.
15. Doyle JR. Extensor tendons: Acute injuries. In: Green DP, Hotchkiss RN, Pederson WC, editors. Green's Operative Hand Surgery. 4th edition. New York: Churchill Livingstone; 1999. p. 195–8.
16. Tubiana R. Mallet finger. In: Tubiana R, editor. Traite de chirurgie de la main. Paris; New York. Masson; 1986. p. 109–21.
17. Abouna JM, Brown H. The treatment of mallet injury. The outcome in a series of 148 consecutive cases and review of the literature. Br J Surg 1968;55:653–67.
18. Gruber JS, Bot AG, Ring D. A prospective randomised controlled trial comparing night splinting with no splinting after treatment of mallet finger. Hand 2014;9:145–50.
19. Alla SR, Deal ND, Dempsey IJ. Current concepts: mallet finger. Hand 2014;9:138–44.
20. Botero S, Hidalgo Diaz JJ, Benaida A, et al. Review of acute traumatic closed mallet finger injuries in adults. Arch Plast Surg 2016;43:134–44.
21. Damron TA, Engber WD. Surgical treatment of mallet finger fractures by tension band technique. Clin Orthop Rel Res 1994;300:133–40.
22. Darder-Pratts A, Fernandez-Garcia E, Fernandez-Garbarder R, et al. Treatment of mallet finger

fractures by the extension-block K-wire technique. J Hand Surg Br 1998;23:802–5.

23. de Jong JP, Nguyen JT, Sonnema AJ, et al. The incidence of acute traumatic tendon injuries in the hand and wrist: a 10-year population-based study. Clin Orthop Surg 2014;6:196–202.

24. Kim JY, Lee SH. Factors related to distal interphalangeal joint extension loss after extension block pinning of mallet finger fractures. J Hand Surg Am 2016;41:414–9.

25. Lin JD, Strauch RJ. Closed soft tissue extensor mechanism injuries (mallet, boutonniere, and saggital band). J Hand Surg Am 2014;39:1005–11.

26. Okafor B, Mbubaegbu C, Munshi I, et al. Mallet deformity of the finger. Five-year follow-up of conservative treatment. J Bone Joint Surg Br 1997;79:544–7.

27. Oflazoglu K, Moradi A, Braun Y, et al. Mallet fractures of the thumb compared with mallet fractures of the fingers. Hand 2017;12:277–82.

28. Osei DA. Clinical research is challenging: commentary on "Factors related to distal interphalangeal joint extension loss after extension block pinning of mallet finger fractures. J Hand Surg Am 2016;41:420–1.

29. Pegoli L, Toh S, Arai K, et al. The Ishiguro extension block technique for the treatment of mallet finger fracture: indications and clinical results. J Hand Surg Eur 2003;28:15–7.

30. Stark HH, Boyes JH, Wilson JN. Mallet finger. J Bone Joint Surg Am 1962;44:1061–8.

31. Vernet P, Igeta Y, Facca S, et al. Treatment of tendinous mallet fingers using a Stack splint versus a dorsal glued splint. Eur J Orth Surg Traum 2019;29:591–6.

The Conservative Treatment of Some Hand and Carpal Fractures

Michel E.H. Boeckstyns, MD, PhD*

KEYWORDS

- Fractures • Hand • Carpal fracture • Conservative treatment

KEY POINTS

- Most fractures of the hand can be managed nonsurgically.
- The trend of treating hand fractures with open reduction and internal fixation must be challenged.
- Almost all fractures of the fifth metacarpal neck and spiral/oblique diaphyseal fractures of the metacarpals can be treated conservatively with a functional brace.
- An alternative to K-wire fixation of base fractures of the proximal phalanges of the fingers is buddy taping to a neighbor finger and immediate mobilization.
- Undisplaced or minimally displaced fractures of the scaphoid—even in the proximal fifth of the bone—can initially be treated by casting and radiological assessment after 6 weeks.

INTRODUCTION

Many—probably most—fractures of the hand can be managed successfully without operation.[1] Nevertheless, in recent decades, there has been a trend toward increased use of operative treatment. The influence of the medical industry and publication bias may have played an important role. During this paradigm shift, it seems that some surgeons have forgotten that a well-functioning hand is more important than a nice-looking radiograph. Open reduction and internal fixation (ORIF) of fractures inevitably carry a risk of surgical complications and this risk often outweighs the advantages of a "perfect" fracture reduction. It may be that some surgeons also deliberately adopt a defensive attitude (defensive medical decision making), by performing ORIF to protect themselves against the patient as a potential plaintiff[2]: if conservative treatment fails to give a perfect result, the patient could claim that operative treatment should have been used while the reverse is less likely to happen.

In the following, I will review some typical fractures that I—based on published evidence and my personal experience—usually treat nonoperatively although the mainstream opinion is that surgery is indicated.

BOXER'S FRACTURE

Many hand surgeons believe that there is an indication for the surgical treatment of neck fractures of the fifth metacarpal in the presence of a dorsal apex angulation or a metacarpal shortening. Some adhere to a cut-off value of 30° for acceptable angulation,[3–7] others to a cut-off value of 40° to 60°.[3,8–21] According to a systematic review of the literature, the dogma that metacarpal neck fractures should be reduced in the presence of angulation exceeding 30° to 40° must be challenged.[22] None of the randomized or quasi-randomized studies that exceeded these threshold values demonstrated any correlation between palmar angulation and the clinical results, which also is supported by other (nonrandomized) studies.[10,23–27] Moreover, the gain of closed reduction before casting is minimal and surgical treatment carries a risk of complications that could be severe.[28] Moreover, the whole issue of fracture

Hand Surgery, Capio PH, Hellerup, Denmark
* Kloeverbakken 11, Virum 2830, Denmark.
E-mail address: mibo@dadlnet.dk

Hand Clin 38 (2022) 289–298
https://doi.org/10.1016/j.hcl.2022.02.001
0749-0712/22/© 2022 Elsevier Inc. All rights reserved.

hand.theclinics.com

angulation is complicated by the fact that measuring dorsal apex angulation is associated with considerable inaccuracy and uncertainty.

Based on my personal experience and the published literature, my preferred treatment of boxer's fracture is nonoperative, using a functional brace for 4 weeks, applied without any attempt at fracture reduction and leaving the fingers free to move, even in the presence of a palmar angulation of 60° to 70° (**Fig. 1**).

In the very rare case of clinically relevant rotational deformity or severe displacement of the metacarpal head, I will perform closed reduction and antegrade (bouquet) percutaneous wiring. In doing so, one must be careful not to fall into the trap of misjudging the apparent malrotation: reduced flexion of the metacarpophalangeal (MCP) joint due to pain may mimic a rotational deformity such that the little finger seeming to be superimposed on the ring finger (**Fig. 2**) although it is not malrotated.

METACARPAL SHAFT FRACTURES

Most single fractures of the metacarpal diaphysis can be treated conservatively.[1,29] There may be a cosmetical advantage of using ORIF but this advantage is outweighed by the higher risk of complications in most instances. The incidence of complications increases with the complexity of the procedure but even with minimal invasive techniques it may be high.[30] The decision as to when surgical treatment is indicated is individual and can be difficult. There are no precise guidelines except that more than minimal malrotation is not acceptable. However, as is the case with metacarpal neck fractures, malrotation is rare because of the derotating action of the intermetacarpal ligaments.[31] In their remarkable prospective study, Kahn and Giddins assessed the outcome of 25 spiral metacarpal fractures treated with early mobilization, even in the presence of malrotation.[31] Twenty-three had excellent outcomes and 2 had good outcomes. Objectively all the fractures united with some shortening of between 2 and 5 mm. Only 2 cases reported mild dysfunction: 1 patient had a residual malrotation of 5° and 1 had some discomfort when boxing. No patients reported any cosmetic problems related to the shortening of the injured fingers. Conservative treatment remains the primary choice for the treatment of spiral or oblique metacarpal fractures. In my hands, it consists of a functional brace and immediate mobilization as described for metacarpal neck fractures. However, it is most important that the patients are instructed carefully in early active exercises. Angulation creating a severe dorsal prominence at the fracture site is an indication for operative treatment. In these cases, I recommend closed reduction and, whenever possible, percutaneous pinning or an intramedullary screw inserted retrograde through the MCP joint.

Plates and screws have very limited or no indications in treating metacarpal fractures. The risk of complications is high,[32–34] although not always appreciated as such. For example, Spies and colleagues[35] concluded that they had a low complication incidence in their series of 38 patients treated with plate and screws or screws alone; however, 3 of the 19 patients who could be reexamined were not satisfied, the mean score of the Disability of the Arm, Shoulder and Hand questionnaire was 41 (24–86) and 5 of the 11 plates had to be removed. Admittedly, other studies do not report such high complication rates[36–38] but safer alternative procedures are available.

PHALANGEAL FRACTURES OF THE FINGERS

Reduction and operative fixation is often indicated for displaced intra-articular fractures. Conversely, many extra-articular fractures can be treated nonoperatively. The maximum benefit of conservative treatment is obtained in those fractures that can be treated with early—sometimes immediate—mobilization. In any case, mobilization of fingers with a diaphyseal phalanx fracture should start as soon as possible and not await radiological consolidation. As a rule, partial active range of motion or intermittent out-of-protection early active motion for a few sessions daily should start within 2 to 3 weeks.[39]

The abduction/hyperextension fracture of the base of the proximal phalanx of the little finger is a common fracture that occurs when the little finger is caught and forcefully pulled ulnarly, often by a dog leash (**Fig. 3**). In children, this mechanism

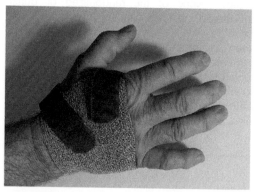

Fig. 1. Functional brace for the treatment of metacarpal fractures.

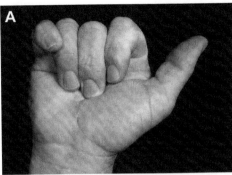
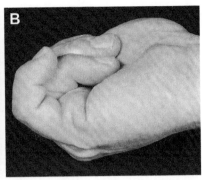

Fig. 2. "Pseudorotational deformity." The little finger seems to be malrotated and scissoring the ring finger. In fact, this is a normal finger, illustrating what happens when stiffness of the metacarpophalangeal joint (in this case faked) prevents normal alignment of the fingers. (A) The little finger overlies the ring finger during flexion of the interphalangeal joints. (B) Lateral view showing the lack of flexion in the metacarpophalangeal joint.

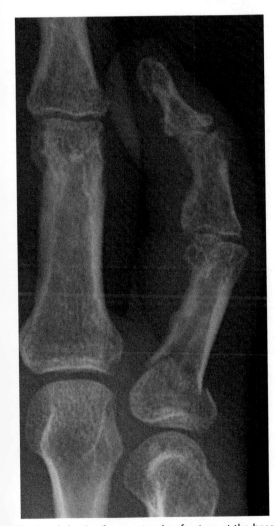

Fig. 3. Abduction/hyperextension fracture at the base of the proximal phalanx of the little finger.

results in a physeal injury (**Fig. 4**). These injuries can be treated successfully with closed reduction, fixation with a single K-wire, and splinting the MCP joint in flexion with mobilization of the proximal interphalangeal joints, until the wire is removed at 24 days and the hand is mobilized freely.[40] However, these fractures can also be treated successfully with closed reduction under local anesthesia, buddy taping to the ring finger, and immediate mobilization. Flexing the finger actively will tend to reduce the dorsal angulation at the fracture site and buddy taping will prevent ulnar deviation. In these cases, it is important to instruct the patients and to check that they perform their exercises properly. Patients who are reluctant to mobilize their fingers must be referred to supervised hand therapy. Radiological reviews are superfluous. Vadstrup and colleagues[41] reported on a prospective cohort of 53 cases, of which 40 could attend a follow-up examination at least 12 months after injury. All fractures united. All but 1 patient regained full flexion of the affected finger to the palm. The mean extension lag was 10° in the proximal interphalangeal joint and 5.5° in the MCP joint. Grip strength returned to normal. Despite these favorable objective findings, 3 patients were dissatisfied by the result because of some swelling, a feeling of stiffness in the fractured finger, or minor functional problems. I have continued using this treatment strategy and have not encountered cases that have complained about a poor result. I find that the main advantage is very fast rehabilitation; the patients are able to resume their usual activities within 4 weeks of their injury (see **Fig. 4**). I have even treated patients with a double fracture, affecting both the little finger and the ring fingers in the same way (**Fig. 5**).

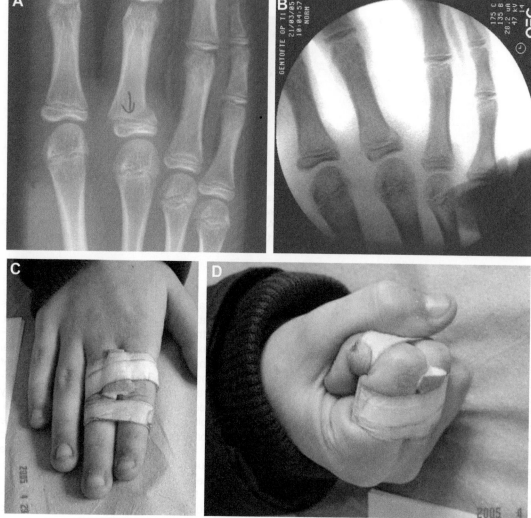

Fig. 4. Physeal injury of the base of the proximal phalanx of the middle finger in a 13-year-old girl. (*A*) Primary radiograph. (*B*) After reduction. (*C, D*) 5 weeks after the injury.

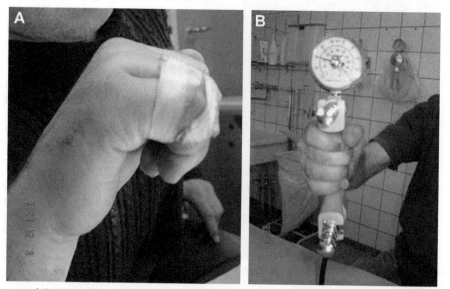

Fig. 5. Fracture of the base of the ring and little fingers. (*A*) Buddy taping after 17 days. (*B*) Functional result after 5 weeks.

SPIRAL AND OBLIQUE FRACTURES OF THE PROXIMAL AND MIDDLE PHALANGES

In contrast to metacarpal fractures, spiral or oblique diaphyseal fractures of the finger phalanges are likely to be unstable and cause clinically important rotational deformity. There may be a remarkable discrepancy between the radiological appearance and the clinical findings (**Fig. 6**). A radiographically displaced oblique fracture of the phalangeal diaphysis with good alignment clinically does not necessarily need internal fixation. In a patient for whom cosmetic issues are not too important, it may be best to accept fracture displacement or simply reduce the deformity under local anesthesia and treat nonoperatively in order to minimize the risk of surgical complications. Conservative treatment is feasible even in the presence of a rotational deformity. Figl and colleagues[42] have reported on the use of functional casting, immobilizing the MCP joints in flexion, and leaving the interphalangeal joints free to move. The authors stress the importance of checking that the patients perform exercises properly, including full extension of the proximal interphalangeal joints.

In my practice, I have found that long spiral fractures of the proximal phalanges, especially in the ring finger, to be particularly challenging and often needing surgical fixation. They may be very unstable and difficult to keep in a correctly reduced position while performing internal or percutaneous fixation. The choice of treatment and the surgery itself should not be delegated to unsupervised junior members of the surgical team or to the occasional hand surgeon. Plate and screw fixation may be tempting but, in my view, this technique should be considered with great care. Despite the advantage of offering stable fixation and thereby the possibility of very early mobilization, there is an increased risk of ending up with reduced mobility due to the increased trauma, stripping of the periosteum, division of a tendon or tendon hood, and the inevitable risk of tendon adhesions; and the surgeon has only "one shot." If after applying the plate, a poor reduction is shown, repositioning of the plate and screws would increase the surgical trauma to an unacceptable level. I therefore advise the more conservative use of closed reduction and 1 or 2 percutaneous K-wires (**Fig. 7**). Local anesthesia is preferable, allowing intraoperative testing of the reduction by having the patient perform active flexion and extension. Fixation with 2 K-wires is more stable so limited range of active finger motion can be started after initial healing of the fracture within the first 2 weeks.[39]

TRANSVERSE FRACTURES OF THE DISTAL PHALANX

Fractures of the distal phalanges are usually transverse, except for avulsion fractures of the tendon attachments. They do not need internal fixation even if displaced. There is no risk of further displacement because of the support of the surrounding soft tissues and the nail. A large gap may need reduction but only fixation if the displacement appears to be unstable. Of course, the Seymour fracture with interposition of the nail bed needs reduction and suture of the wound but supplementary K-wire fixation is mostly superfluous.

SCAPHOID FRACTURES

There is an increasing trend to treat undisplaced or minimally displaced waist fractures of the scaphoid with screw fixation rather than nonoperatively with immobilization in a plaster cast. The main argument for treating them operatively is that it shortens return to work and time to union without a significant difference in the incidence of complications as concluded in the systematic review by Alnaeem and colleagues.[43] In particular,

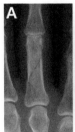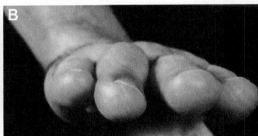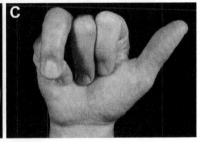

Fig. 6. Spiral fracture of the proximal phalanx of the ring finger. (*A*) Radiologically this fracture seems undisplaced. (*B, C*) Clinically there is a malrotation of about 25° causing scissoring of the ring and little fingers. (*From* Boeckstyns MEH. Current methods, outcomes and challenges for the treatment of hand fractures. J Hand Surg Eur 2020;45(6):547-559 with permission.)

percutaneous or minimally invasive fracture fixation seems to yield faster rehabilitation[44]; however, there is no consensus. Several high-quality studies have found a higher complication incidence after operative treatment.[45–48] These complications include infection, poor placement of the screw with damage of cartilage, chronic regional pain syndrome, scar problems, and osteoarthritis of the scaphotrapeziotrapezoidal joint. In the SWIFT study,[47] 219 minimally displaced (<2 mm) scaphoid waist fractures were randomly assigned to screw fixation while 220 were treated with a cast. Besides 4 cases with numbness of the scar area or decreased sensation on the dorsum of the hand, complications after surgery included 2 infections, 1 case of complex regional pain syndrome and 8 cases that had a reoperation for removal of a protruding screw. Conversely, the cast group had 1 transient nerve problem, 2 infections, no complex regional pain syndrome, and only 1 reoperation due to nonunion. The duration of sick leave was similar in the 2 groups. Some studies even fail to reveal a significant shorter return to work time after operative treatment of scaphoid waist fractures.[44,46]

Thus, the general advice for waist fractures is to discuss the pros and cons of surgical and nonsurgical treatment with the patients or to adopt a so-called aggressive conservative treatment with initial cast immobilization, careful assessment of fracture healing with radiographs and computed tomographic (CT) scans if necessary, after 6 to 8 weeks of cast immobilization and recommending surgical fixation with or without bone grafting at that time if a gap is identified at the fracture site. Usually, the scaphoid can then be fixed with a percutaneous screw. Such an approach should result in fracture union incidence over 95%.[46]

Proximal pole fractures, defined as fractures in the proximal one-fifth of the bone, have a much higher incidence of nonunion than waist fractures if treated nonoperatively. The relative risk of nonunion is 7.5 compared with more distal fractures according to the meta-analysis of Eastley and colleagues.[49] Consequently, operative treatment is generally advised even for nondisplaced or minimally displaced proximal pole fractures. On the webpage AO Surgery Reference, it is stated that prograde screw fixation is indicated for "virtually all proximal pole scaphoid fractures… The only contraindication is low functional demand patients." It also states that "Nonoperative treatment requires a prolonged period of plaster immobilization (3–6 months)." But not all studies report a nonunion incidence (10%) that is significantly higher than after surgical treatment.[50]

Personally, I challenge the general recommendation of surgical treatment of all proximal pole fractures, including undisplaced or minimally displaced, and agree with the views of Johnson and Dias.[51] There is no conclusive evidence that initial surgical treatment produces better ultimate results, surgery is costly, and unnecessary use of operation theater time could be avoided. "Injudicious operative treatment of scaphoid fractures can lead to disastrous outcomes that may not be

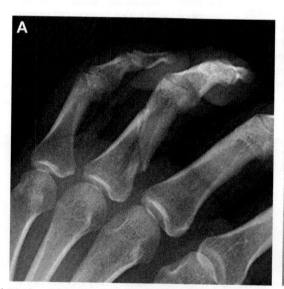
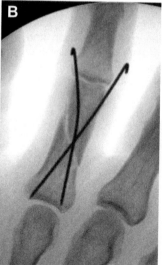

Fig. 7. (*A*) Displaced fracture of the proximal phalanx. (*B*) This fracture could have been treated nonoperatively but the clinical deformity was not acceptable for the patient and K-wire fixation was performed. (*Courtesy of* Dr. Silvia Stierle, MD, North Norway University, Tromsoe, Norway.)

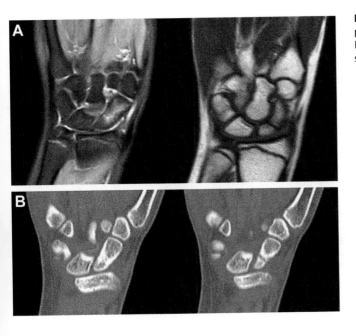

Fig. 8. 16-year-old girl with undisplaced proximal scaphoid fracture. (*A*) Initial MRI. (*B*) CT scan after 6 weeks in cast showing partial healing.

remedied."[52] My strategy in cases without an increased risk of complications (young, healthy, compliant, nonsmoking patients presenting early) is "aggressive conservative treatment," assessing the progression of union with CT scans after 6 to 8 weeks (**Fig. 8**). If there is no evidence of partial (ie, at least 50%) union at that time, I advise immediate percutaneous screw fixation. If the CT scans reveal cystic degeneration of the fracture site, I would use arthroscopically assisted cancellous bone grafting from the distal radius and screw fixation.[53] Conversely, if there is ongoing consolidation of the fracture, I will continue conservative treatment for another 2 to 4 weeks and check again radiographically. I consider that more than half of the patients can avoid surgery with this strategy. The disadvantage of this strategy is a prolonged period of immobilization (additional 4–6 weeks) for some patients but the cost-benefit balance of a prolonged sick leave versus increased costs for surgical complications is difficult to assess. The final choice of treatment will always be based on shared decision making with the patient.

HAND THERAPY

Hand therapy is a very important component of the team treating hand fractures. It certainly has saved the mobility of many fingers after complex fractures treated with ORIF. However, with conservative treatment as proposed earlier, hand therapy is often unnecessary. The key is to mobilize as early as possible and avoid immobilization of joints that do not need immobilizing. It is most important to educate patients carefully and check that they have understood and can perform the exercises they have been instructed. This may require extra clinic appointments. I recommend you do not apply a buddy tape and send the patient home without being sure they will perform adequate mobilization of their fingers. Pain may prevent a full range of motion of the free joints but it should diminish within a few days and in the meanwhile, the fingers must be moved as much as pain allows. Every day without motion will cause the pain to return again and again. In my practice, supervised hand therapy is only indicated in rare instances of marked swelling and stiffness especially if heading toward complex regional pain syndrome.

SUMMARY

The most important goal when treating a fracture of the hand is to preserve functional alignment and mobility of the fingers. A good cosmetic result is also important, more for some people than for others. ORIF may correct alignment better than conservative treatment but the price can be reduced mobility or more disastrous complications. Conversely, unnecessary prolonged immobilization when treating fractures nonoperatively also can lead to troublesome stiffness.

Too often the decision on how to treat a hand fracture is delegated to less experienced doctors. The decision whether to operate or not may be difficult and requires considerable experience. It may depend on many factors including the patient's needs, age, profession and leisure activities, and the surgeon's preference and experience.

Textbooks may give indications but true evidence covering all types of fractures and their subgroups is usually lacking and, if available, reports can be contradictory. Moreover, favorable results of surgery are probably over-represented, leading to a heightened belief in the superiority of surgical techniques.

This article reports some fracture types and subtypes that are increasingly treated surgically but mostly can be managed by conservative means." Defining fracture patterns and subgroups and conducting prospective studies is essential....national or international evidence-based guidelines must be set out for as many fracture types as possible, not only for the large diagnostic groups."[29] Continuous education of younger hand surgeons is equally important.

CLINICS CARE POINTS

- Operative treatment of hand fractures carries a risk of increased complication incidence.

- Before embarking in operative treatment, the possibility of safe conservative treatment should be considered.

- Fracture union with a minor deformity is usually well-tolerated.

- Whenever possible, fractures fingers should be carefully mobilized within 2 to 3 weeks without awaiting radiological consolidation.

DISCLOSURE

The author has nothing to disclose.

REFERENCES

1. Giddins GE. The non-operative management of hand fractures. J Hand Surg Eur 2015;40:33–41.
2. Boeckstyns MEH. Clinical decision making in hand surgery. J Hand Surg Eur 2018;43:568–70.
3. Kim JK, Kim DJ. Antegrade intramedullary pinning versus retrograde intramedullary pinning for displaced fifth metacarpal neck fractures. Clin Orthop Relat Res 2015;473:1747–54.
4. Surke C, Meier R, Haug L, et al. Osteosynthesis of fifth metacarpal neck fractures with a photodynamic polymer bone stabilization system. J Hand Surg Eur 2020;45:119–25.
5. Tank P, Patel V, Ninama D. A prospective study of 15 cases of fifth metacarpal neck fractures treated by antegrade single blunt-tip k wire: Surgical technique, clinico-radiological outcome. Nat J Clin Orthop 2018;2:30–4.
6. Winter M, Balaguer T, Bessiere C, et al. Surgical treatment of the boxer's fracture: transverse pinning versus intramedullary pinning. J Hand Surg Eur 2007;32:709–13.
7. Wong KP, Hay RA, Tay SC. Surgical outcomes of fifth metacarpal neck fractures–a comparative analysis of dorsal plating versus tension band wiring. Hand Surg 2015;20:99–105.
8. Cepni SK, Aykut S, Bekmezci T, et al. A minimally invasive fixation technique for selected patients with fifth metacarpal neck fracture. Injury 2016;47: 1270–5.
9. Chen KJ, Wang JP, Yin CY, et al. Fixation of fifth metacarpal neck fractures: a comparison of medial locking plates with intramedullary K-wires. J Hand Surg Eur 2020;45:567–73.
10. Eldridge J, Apau D. Boxer's fracture: management and outcomes. Emerg Nurse 2015;23:24–30.
11. Elmowafy H, Elsaedy A, Hassan A. Bouquet technique in the treatment of metacarpal fractures. Menoufia Med J 2018;31:1312–6.
12. Facca S, Ramdhian R, Pelissier A, et al. Fifth metacarpal neck fracture fixation: Locking plate versus K-wire? Orthop Traumatol Surg Res 2010;96:506–12.
13. Fujitani R, Omokawa S, Shigematsu K, et al. Comparison of the intramedullary nail and low-profile plate for unstable metacarpal neck fractures. J Orthop Sci 2012;17:450–6.
14. Kaynak G, Botanlioglu H, Caliskan M, et al. Comparison of functional metacarpal splint and ulnar gutter splint in the treatment of fifth metacarpal neck fractures: a prospective comparative study. BMC Musculoskelet Disord 2019;20:169.
15. Ozturk I, Erturer E, Sahin F, et al. Effects of fusion angle on functional results following non-operative treatment for fracture of the neck of the fifth metacarpal. Injury 2008;39:1464–6.
16. Pogliacomi F, Mijno E, Pedrazzini A, et al. Fifth metacarpal neck fractures: fixation with antegrade locked flexible intramedullary nailing. Acta Biomed 2017; 88:57–64.
17. Potenza V, Caterini R, De Maio F, et al. Fractures of the neck of the fifth metacarpal bone. Medium-term results in 28 cases treated by percutaneous transverse pinning. Injury 2012;43:242–5.
18. Poumellec MA, Dreant N. Elastic retrograde intramedullary percutaneous pinning for fifth metacarpal neck fractures: a series of 32 patients. Hand Surg Rehabil 2017;36:250–4.
19. Rhee SH, Lee SK, Lee SL, et al. Prospective multicenter trial of modified retrograde percutaneous intramedullary Kirschner wire fixation for displaced metacarpal neck and shaft fractures. Plast Reconstr Surg 2012;129:694–703.

20. Sadiq M, Hussain S. Management of boxers fracture with single antegrade bent K-wire. Inter J Res Orthop 2019;5:398–402.

21. She Y, Xu Y. Treatment of fifth metacarpal neck fractures with antegrade single elastic intramedullary nailing. BMC Musculoskelet Disord 2017;18:238.

22. Boeckstyns MEH. Challenging the dogma: severely angulated neck fractures of the fifth metacarpal must be treated surgically. J Hand Surg Eur 2021; 46:30–6.

23. Arafa M, Haines J, Noble J, et al. Immediate mobilization of fractures of the neck of the fifth metacarpal. Injury 1986;17:277–8.

24. Braakman M, Oderwald EE, Haentjens MH. Functional taping of fractures of the 5th metacarpal results in a quicker recovery. Injury 1998;29:5–9.

25. Ford DJ, Ali MS, Steel WM. Fractures of the fifth metacarpal neck: is reduction or immobilisation necessary? J Hand Surg Br 1989;14:165–7.

26. Hansen PB, Hansen TB. The treatment of fractures of the ring and little metacarpal necks. A prospective randomized study of three different types of treatment. J Hand Surg Br 1998;23:245–7.

27. Westbrook AP, Davis TR, Armstrong D, et al. The clinical significance of malunion of fractures of the neck and shaft of the little finger metacarpal. J Hand Surg Eur 2008;33:732–9.

28. Sletten IN, Hellund JC, Olsen B, et al. Conservative treatment has comparable outcome with bouquet pinning of little finger metacarpal neck fractures: a multicentre randomized controlled study of 85 patients. J Hand Surg Eur 2015;40:76–83.

29. Boeckstyns MEH. Current methods, outcomes and challenges for the treatment of hand fractures. J Hand Surg Eur 2020;45:547–59.

30. Dumont C, Burchhardt H, Tezval M. [Soft tissue protective and minimally invasive osteosynthesis for metacarpal fractures II-V]. Oper Orthop Traumatol 2012;24:312–23.

31. Khan A, Giddins G. The outcome of conservative treatment of spiral metacarpal fractures and the role of the deep transverse metacarpal ligaments in stabilizing these injuries. J Hand Surg Eur 2015; 40:59–62.

32. Fusetti C, Meyer H, Borisch N, et al. Complications of plate fixation in metacarpal fractures. J Trauma 2002;52:535–9.

33. Soni A, Gulati A, Bassi JL, et al. Outcome of closed ipsilateral metacarpal fractures treated with mini fragment plates and screws: a prospective study. J Orthop Traumatol 2012;13:29–33.

34. Page SM, Stern PJ. Complications and range of motion following plate fixation of metacarpal and phalangeal fractures. J Hand Surg Am 1998;23: 827–32.

35. Spies CK, Langer M, Hohendorff B, et al. [Open reduction and screw/plate osteosynthesis of metacarpal fractures]. Oper Orthop Traumatol 2019;31:422–32.

36. Baumgartner RE, Federer AE, Guerrero EM, et al. Complications of low-profile plate fixation in metacarpal fractures. Orthopedics 2021;44:e91–4.

37. Dreyfuss D, Allon R, Izacson N, et al. A comparison of locking plates and intramedullary pinning for fixation of metacarpal shaft fractures. Hand (N Y) 2019; 14:27–33.

38. Ahmed Z, Haider MI, Buzdar MI, et al. Comparison of miniplate and K-wire in the treatment of metacarpal and phalangeal fractures. Cureus 2020;12:e7039.

39. Tang JB. Efficient and elaborate treatment of hand fractures. J Hand Surg Eur 2015;40:7.

40. Shewring DJ, Trickett RW, Smith A. Fractures at the junction of diaphysis and metaphysis of the proximal phalanges in adults. J Hand Surg Eur 2018;43: 506–12.

41. Vadstrup LS, Jorring S, Bernt P, et al. Base fractures of the fifth proximal phalanx can be treated conservatively with buddy taping and immediate mobilisation. Dan Med J 2014;61:A4882.

42. Figl M, Weninger P, Hofbauer M, et al. Results of dynamic treatment of fractures of the proximal phalanx of the hand. J Trauma 2011;70:852–6.

43. Alnaeem H, Aldekhayel S, Kanevsky J, et al. A systematic review and meta-analysis examining the differences between nonsurgical management and percutaneous fixation of minimally and nondisplaced scaphoid fractures. J Hand Surg Am 2016; 41:1135–11344 e1.

44. Li H, Guo W, Guo S, et al. Surgical versus nonsurgical treatment for scaphoid waist fracture with slight or no displacement: a meta-analysis and systematic review. Medicine (Baltimore) 2018;97:e13266.

45. Clementson M, Jorgsholm P, Besjakov J, et al. Conservative treatment versus arthroscopic-assisted screw fixation of scaphoid waist fractures–a randomized trial with minimum 4-year follow-up. J Hand Surg Am 2015;40:1341–8.

46. Dias JJ, Wildin CJ, Bhowal B, et al. Should acute scaphoid fractures be fixed? A randomized controlled trial. J Bone Joint Surg Am 2005;87: 2160–8.

47. Dias JJ, Brealey SD, Fairhurst C, et al. Surgery versus cast immobilisation for adults with a bicortical fracture of the scaphoid waist (SWIFFT): a pragmatic, multicentre, open-label, randomised superiority trial. Lancet 2020;396(10248):390–401.

48. Vinnars B, Pietreanu M, Bodestedt A, et al. Nonoperative compared with operative treatment of acute scaphoid fractures. A randomized clinical trial. J Bone Joint Surg Am 2008;90:1176–85.

49. Eastley N, Singh H, Dias JJ, et al. Union rates after proximal scaphoid fractures; meta-analyses and review of available evidence. J Hand Surg Eur 2013; 38:888–97.

50. Grewal R, Lutz K, MacDermid JC, et al. Proximal Pole Scaphoid Fractures: a Computed Tomographic Assessment of Outcomes. J Hand Surg Am 2016; 41:54–8.

51. Johnson NA, Morris H, Dias JJ. Questions regarding the evidence guiding treatment of displaced scaphoid fractures. J Hand Surg Eur 2021;46:213–8.

52. Kawamura K, Chung KC. Treatment of scaphoid fractures and nonunions. J Hand Surg Am 2008; 33:988–97.

53. Wang JP, Huang HK, Shih JT. Arthroscopic-assisted reduction, bone grafting and screw fixation across the scapholunate joint for proximal pole scaphoid nonunion. BMC Musculoskelet Disord 2020;21:834.

Internal Fixation of Finger Fractures
Field Sterility for Surgery and Earlier Removal of K-Wires Are Safe

Donald Lalonde, MD, FRCSC[a],*, Colton Boudreau, MD[b]

KEYWORDS

- Early protected movement • Finger fracture • WALANT • Early K wire removal at 2 to 3 weeks
- Clinical healing of finger/hand fractures • Field sterility for K wire insertion

KEY POINTS

- There is no increase in infection rates when K-wire insertion is performed with field sterility.
- K-wires are better removed early at 2 to 4 weeks when there is clinical healing.
- Fractures are clinically healed when there is no pain to firm palpation of the fracture site.
- Radiographic healing of finger fractures is not as valuable as clinical healing.
- WALANT lets surgeons assess the stability of K-wire fixation with full fist flexion and extension testing during surgery.

INTRODUCTION

Field sterility for K-wire insertion outside the main operating room (OR) is much cheaper and greener, that is, there is less waste. It permits increased access to more affordable surgery because unnecessary sedation and full sterility are eliminated. There is no increase in infection rates when K-wire insertion is performed with field sterility.

USEFULNESS OF K-WIRE FIXATION AND EARLY PROTECTED MOVEMENT

Background of Usefulness of K-Wire Fixation and Early Protected Movement in Hand and Finger Fractures

Why is percutaneous closed reduction and fixation with K-wires still popular? Less dissection means less postoperative scarring and stiffness

Many senior surgeons like the author D.L. started their career with K-wire or interosseus wire fixation, then moved to plates and screws when they were developed for the hand in the 1980s, then moved back to K-wires to get better results. Percutaneous closed K-wire fixation is a very effective method of treating unstable finger fractures. Less dissection leads to less scarring and less callus formation. This in turn can lead to less stiffness and shorter rehabilitation time if it is combined with early protected movement.

Although there are complications with K-wires,[1] there is good high-level evidence that plate and screw fixation with wide dissection is not superior to K-wires, even without early protected movement of the K-wired groups.[2–8] Plate fixation also has complications including frequently requiring removal at a second operation.[9,10] Although much more expensive, minimally invasive intramedullary screw fixation may be a good alternative to K-wires if future long-term studies show no increase in arthritis from screw placement via joints[11]

[a] Surgery, Division of Plastic Surgery, Dalhousie University, Suite C204, 600 Main Street, Saint John, New Brunswick E2K 1J5, Canada; [b] Division of Plastic Surgery, Dalhousie University, 6016 Pepperell Street, Apartment 508, Halifax, Nova Scotia B3J0C6, Canada
* Corresponding author.
E-mail address: dlalonde@drlalonde.ca

Hand Clin 38 (2022) 299–303
https://doi.org/10.1016/j.hcl.2022.02.002
0749-0712/22/© 2022 Elsevier Inc. All rights reserved.

*Early protected movement of K-wired finger
fractures is good; rigid fixation is not required
for pain-guided early protected movement*

Hand and finger fractures stabilized with K-wires
are traditionally immobilized for 4 weeks or
more.[12] Just like in flexor tendon repair, early protected movement of K-wire fixed finger fractures at
3 to 5 days after surgery can lead to better outcomes.[13,14] Rigid internal fixation of finger fractures is not required for pain-guided early
protected movement protocols. If patients do not
do what hurts, they are not likely to lose their
reduction or get infections around the K-wires.[15]

Wide awake K-wire fixation allows the surgeon
to see a patient move their K-wired finger fracture
through full fist flexion and extension at the end of
the operation. The surgeon then knows that his
K-wires are stable enough that the patient can
make half a fist when the swelling starts to subside
a few days postoperatively, so the tendons do not
get stuck in the scar with prolonged immobilization. The surgeon knows that moving the K-wired
finger a little will not disrupt the fracture reduction.

Three Reasons Why We Should Move K-Wire Fixation of Hand and Finger Fractures Out of the Main OR and into Minor Procedure Rooms.

*Field sterility for K-wiring finger fractures has
the same infection rate as full main OR sterility*

Evidence-based field sterility[16] means that the surgeon wears sterile gloves and a mask. There is no
head cover or gown. There does not need to be a
special ventilation system in the room. Field sterility
means that only the part of the body undergoing surgery needs to be sterilized. For K-wiring of fingers,
that means that only the hand and wrist are sterilized
and draped. The part of the x-ray device involved in
the K-wiring also becomes part of the sterile field
with sterile towels or a sterile cover (**Fig. 1**).

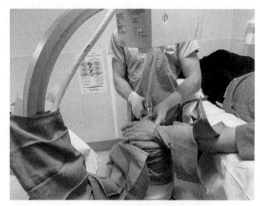

Fig. 1. Field sterility for K-wire insertion has the same
infection rate as main OR full sterility.

For many years, Canadians have been using
field sterility for carpal tunnel surgery and K-wire
fixation of finger fractures with acceptably low
infection rates.[17] Many centers have reported
very low infection rates with field sterility insertion
of K-wires for finger fractures and other minor
hand surgery procedures[18–25] In addition to the
evidence data from those studies, we are in the
process of publishing a study of more than 1050
patients from a multicenter (19 cities), prospective,
Canadian trial comparing full OR sterility to minor
procedure room sterility for percutaneous K-wiring
of finger fractures with no significant difference in
infection rates (personal communication).

*Field sterility is much less expensive because it
avoids unnecessary personnel, draping, and
supplies that are part of routine main OR
procedures*

Most main ORs are required to have at least 2
nurses in the room, even if the procedure is performed under local anesthesia alone. Many operating theaters insist that patients have some
sedation, whether they need it or not. The
personnel required for this are very costly. We
only have one nurse to help the surgeon do the
surgery with field sterility, and no recovery room
personnel are required. Patients sit up and go
home like they have been to the dentist for a filling.

Most main ORs open large bundles of sterile
supplies and drapes that are not necessary for
K-wire surgery. Many of these supplies are never
used, do not decrease infection rates, and end
up in unnecessary medical waste that pollutes
our land and waters.[26,27]

*Field sterility WALANT K-wire insertion in
procedure rooms outside of the main OR will
greatly improve access to corrective surgery for
those who cannot currently afford unnecessary
sedation and full main OR sterility*

Many patients in developing countries go onto
malunion and stiffness after finger fractures
because they cannot afford unnecessary sedation
and full OR sterility for K-wire insertion. Moving
these procedures into minor procedure rooms as
we have in Canada will make fracture fixation
much more accessible to the poor of the
world.[28,29]

EARLY REMOVAL OF K-WIRES AT 2 TO 3 WEEKS AFTER PINNING
Clinical Healing of Finger Fractures is Much More Useful Than Radiological Healing

In the case in **Fig. 2**, the patient presented to the
senior author with a 2-month-old malunited finger
fracture with scissoring. Radiographs were

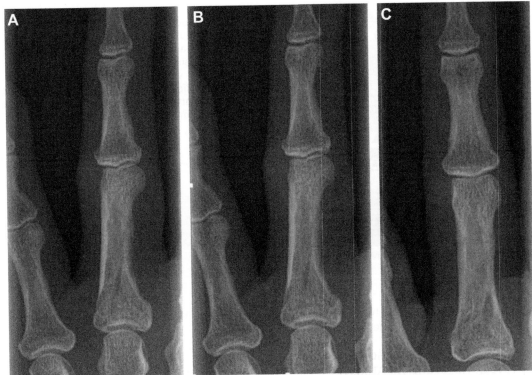

Fig. 2. Two-month-old scissoring malunited fracture. X-rays interpreted by radiologist as "osseus union not complete" when fracture healing was found to be rock solid at the time of surgery. (*A*) Lateral view, (*B, C*) Oblique and posterior-anterior views.

interpreted by a radiologist as "osseus union not complete". When we palpated the fracture site with firm pressure, there was zero pain. No pain on fracture palpation means the fracture is clinically healed and will be impossible to reduce without opening the fracture and chiseling out the callus, or performing an osteotomy, which is what we had to do in this case. Surgeons see this all the time; radiologists state that finger fractures are not healed, but they are "solid as rock" when we operate on them.

Earlier Removal of K-Wires at 2 to 3 Weeks is Safe When the Fracture is Clinically Healed (No Pain on Palpation)

Most K-wires are traditionally removed from hand fractures at 4 to 6 weeks after insertion.[30] For many years in our city, we have routinely removed K-wires when the fractures were clinically healed at 2 to 3 weeks with no pain to palpation of the fracture site (as above).[31] Earlier removal of K-wires and early protected movement frequently provide us a full range of motion of a K-wired finger fracture by 4 weeks when traditionally treated immobilized K-wired fingers are just coming out of a plaster cast. See **Fig. 3** for a typically

managed K-wired finger in a reliable patient in our practice.

When to be Careful About When Removing K-Wires Early at 2 to 3 Weeks After Insertion, Even with Apparent Clinical Healing (No Pain to Firm Palpation of the Fracture Site)

When there is a good blood supply, as in younger patients, K-wires can be safely removed as early as 10 days in some cases. However, if the blood supply is less good, or if sensation is lacking, healing is slower making clinical assessment of healing less reliable, and waiting 4 weeks or longer may be wise. Examples of slower healing with less blood supply or diminished sensation are as follows: (1) operative stripping of periosteal blood supply when a fracture has to be opened, as opposed to a "preserved" blood supply with closed reduction; (2) wood splitter injuries where the periosteal blood supply is degloved off of the bone by the wood splitter; (3) older patients with renal failure, poor sensation and poor capillary refill of the fingertips; (4) patients who have altered pain sensation, for example, because they are on chronic pain killers and cannot accurately know what hurts; and (5) numb fingers with nerve injuries

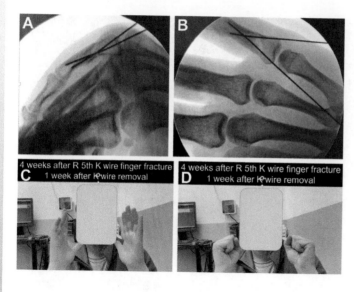

Fig. 3. (*A, B*) K-wires in place after closed reduction of a right 5th finger proximal phalanx fracture with an incidental old, healed mallet fracture (*C, D*) showing result of finger extension and flexion 4 weeks after K-wiring with pain-guided early protected movement started 4 days after surgery and K-wires removed at 3 weeks after surgery.

where determination of clinical healing with pain on palpation is much less reliable.

SUMMARY: ACHIEVING THE GOALS OF HAND AND FINGER FRACTURE TREATMENT

The main goals of hand and finger fracture management are a pain-free full or nearly range of motion with no scissoring. The biggest problem we all face is stiffness. Two of the main reasons for stiffness are prolonged immobilization and excessive surgical dissection that leads to increased internal scarring and adhesions. Minimally invasive percutaneous K-wiring in an affordable environment with early protected movement and early K-wire removal contribute to a reduction in stiffness and a more rapid return to normal hand function.

DISCLOSURE

The authors have nothing to disclose.

REFERENCES

1. Stahl S, Schwartz O. Complications of K-wire fixation of fractures and dislocations in the hand and wrist. Arch Orthop Trauma Surg 2001;121:527–30.
2. Facca S, Ramdhian R, Pelissier A, et al. Fifth metacarpal neck fracture fixation: locking plate versus K-wire? Orthop Traumatol Surg Res 2010;96:506–12.
3. Ahmed Z, Haider MI, Buzdar MI, et al. Comparison of miniplate and K-wire in the treatment of metacarpal and phalangeal fractures. Cureus 2020; 12(2):e7039.
4. Greeven AP, Bezstarosti S, Krijnen P, et al. Open reduction and internal fixation versus percutaneous transverse Kirschner wire fixation for single, closed second to fifth metacarpal shaft fractures: a systematic review. Eur J Trauma Emerg Surg 2016;42: 169–75.
5. Melamed E, Joo L, Lin E, et al. Plate fixation versus percutaneous pinning for unstable metacarpal fractures: a meta-analysis. J Hand Surg Asian Pac 2017; 22:29–34.
6. Bao B, Zhu H, Zheng X. Plate versus Kirschner wire fixation in treatment of fourth and fifth carpometacarpal fracture-dislocations: a retrospective cohort study. Int J Surg 2018;52:293–6.
7. Pasquino A, Tomarchio A, De Cruto E, et al. Comparing hand strength and quality life of locking plate versus intramedullary K wire for transverse midshaft metacarpal fractures. Med Glas (Zenica) 2021;18:316–21.
8. Reformat DD, Nores GG, Lam G, et al. outcome analysis of metacarpal and phalangeal fixation techniques at Bellevue Hospital. Ann Plast Surg 2018;81:407–10.
9. Chen KJ, Wang JP, Yin CY, et al. Fixation of fifth metacarpal neck fractures: a comparison of medial locking plates with intramedullary K-wires. J Hand Surg Eur 2020;45:567–73.
10. Hay RA, Tay SC. A comparison of K-wire versus screw fixation on the outcomes of distal phalanx fractures. J Hand Surg Am 2015;40:2160–7.
11. Brewer CF, Young-Sing Q, Sierakowski A. cost comparison of Kirschner wire versus intramedullary screw fixation of metacarpal and phalangeal fractures. Hand (N Y) 2021. https://doi.org/10.1177/15589447211030690. 15589447211030690.
12. Vasilakis V, Sinnott CJ, Hamade M, et al. Extra-articular metacarpal fractures: closed reduction and percutaneous pinning versus open reduction and internal fixation. Plast Reconstr Surg Glob Open 2019; 7(5):e2261.

13. Gregory S, Lalonde DH, Fung Leung LT. Minimally invasive finger fracture management: wide-awake closed reduction, K-wire fixation, and early protected movement. Hand Clin 2014;30:7–15.

14. Mohammed R, Farook MZ, Newman K. Percutaneous elastic intramedullary nailing of metacarpal fractures: surgical technique and clinical results study. J Orthop Surg Res 2011;6:37.

15. Lalonde D. Finger Fractures. In: Lalonde D, editor. Wide awake hand surgery. Newyork: Thieme; 2016. p. 237–64.

16. Yu J, Ji T, Craig M, et al. Evidence-based sterility: The evolving role of field sterility in skin and minor hand surgery. Plast Reconstr Surg Glob Open 2019;7(11):e2481.

17. Leblanc MR, Lalonde DH, Thoma A, et al. Is main operating room sterility really necessary in carpal tunnel surgery? A multicenter prospective study of minor procedure room field sterility surgery. Hand (N Y). 2011;6:60–3.

18. Dua K, Blevins CJ, O'Hara NN, et al. The safety and benefits of the semisterile technique for closed reduction and percutaneous pinning of pediatric upper extremity fractures. Hand (N Y) 2019;14:808–13.

19. Garon MT, Massey P, Chen A, et al. Cost and complications of percutaneous fixation of hand fractures in a procedure room versus the operating room. Hand (N Y). 2018;13:428–34.

20. Jagodzinski NA, Ibish S, Furniss D. Surgical site infection after hand surgery outside the operating theatre: a systematic review. J Hand Surg Eur 2017;42:289–94.

21. Steve AK, Schrag CH, Kuo A, et al. metacarpal fracture fixation in a minor surgery setting versus main operating room: a cost-minimization analysis. Plast Reconstr Surg Glob Open 2019;7:e2298.

22. Starker I, Eaton RG. Kirschner wire placement in the emergency room. Is there a risk? J Hand Surg Br 1995;20:535–8.

23. Hashemi K, Blakeley CJ. Wound infections in daycase hand surgery: a prospective study. Ann R Coll Surg Engl 2004;86:449–50.

24. Halvorson AJ, Sechriest VF 2nd, Gravely A, et al. Risk of surgical site infection after carpal tunnel release performed in an operating room versus a clinic-based procedure room within a Veterans Affairs Medical Center. Am J Infect Control 2020;48: 173–7.

25. Avoricani A, Dar Q-A, Levy KH, et al. WALANT hand and upper extremity procedures performed with minor field sterility are associated with low infection rates. Plasit Surg (Oakv) 2022;30:122–9.

26. Bravo D, Gaston RG, Melamed E. Environmentally responsible hand surgery: past, present, and future. J Hand Surg Am 2020;45:444–8.

27. Van Demark RE Jr, Smith VJS, Fiegen A. Lean and Green Hand Surgery. J Hand Surg Am 2018;43: 179–81.

28. Behar BJ, Danso OO, Farhart B, et al. Collaboration in outreach: The Kumasi, Ghana model. Hand Clin 2019;35:429–34.

29. Holoyda KA, Farhat B, Lalonde DH, et al. Creating an outpatient, local anesthetic hand operating room in a resource-constrained Ghanaian hospital builds surgical capacity and financial stability. Ann Plast Surg 2020;84:385–9.

30. Boussakri H, Elidrissi M, Azarkane M, et al. Fractures of the neck of the fifth metacarpal bone, treated by percutaneous intramedullary nailing: surgical technique, radiological and clinical results study (28 cases). Pan Afr Med J 2014;18:187.

31. Lalonde D. Preferred methods that go against traditional teachings. J Hand Sur Eur 2021;46:327–30.

The Trapezium is Not Necessary
Logical Implications in Treating Basal Joint Arthritis and Pollicization

Ulrich Mennen, MBChB(Pret), FRCS(Glasg), FRCS(Edin), FCS(SA)
Orth, MMed(Orth), FHMVS(DUMC), MD(Orth), DSc(Med)*

KEYWORDS

- Trapezium • Osteoarthritis • First carpometacarpal joint • Base of thumb arthritis • Pollicization
- Thumb ligament reconstruction • Ball-and-socket joint

KEY POINTS

- A ball-and-socket joint is inherently stable. As the thumb needs to be stable in many directions, this mechanical type of joint is the most classic to provide both stability and mobility at the same time.
- Therefore, a simple excision of the trapezium for osteoarthritis of the base of thumb joint gives the ultimate functional stability and mobility.
- Ligamentous reconstruction is thus also not necessary because of the obvious mechanical stability. If left undisturbed, the subperiosteal released ligaments will reattach themselves during the healing process and only act to limit excessive mobility of the thumb.
- Any kind of material inserted into the socket created by removing the trapezium will interfere with the stability of the thumb. This is the most logical concept that has been stubbornly ignored!
- The same principles as above apply if a pollicization is performed.

INTRODUCTION

The thumb carpometacarpal or trapeziometacarpal-1 (TMC1) joint allows multidirectional movements, while being amazingly stable for the forces exerted on it in pinch and grip. Because this joint is subjected to large and constant mechanical demands, it is also prone to degeneration over time, commonly causing not only pain and functional loss but also an unacceptable cosmetic appearance. It has long been thought that the mechanics of this joint had to be replicated when diseased. Innumerable surgical and nonsurgical methods have been proposed, tried, published, and often abandoned relatively quickly. The literature is vast reporting various stabilizing methods, tissue and artificial prostheses, and serious complications attempting to mimic the impossibly complex biomechanics. Most of these procedures have been discarded because of failures of the artificial reconstructions or complications because of the inherent lack of understanding the very complicated and intricate forces exerted on this joint.

The aim of this article is to discuss the outcomes of the author's practice in a large series of simple trapezium excision for the painful degenerative TMC1 joint. My outcomes indicate simple treatment method is sufficient and that any interposition and ligamentous reconstruction is unnecessary. This observation has previously been confirmed by many other researchers.[1]

ANATOMY OF THE TRAPEZIOMETACARPAL-1 JOINT

The TMC1 joint allows the thumb to flex, extend, abduct, adduct, and rotate. A combination of

University of Pretoria and Jacaranda Hospital, Pretoria, South Africa. Editor IFSSH Ezine.
* 7 Siskin Avenue, Chapman's Bay Estate, Noordhoek, Cape Town 7979, South Africa.
E-mail address: ulrichmennen@gmail.com
Website: http://www.ulrichmennen.co.za

Hand Clin 38 (2022) 305–312
https://doi.org/10.1016/j.hcl.2022.02.007
0749-0712/22/© 2022 Elsevier Inc. All rights reserved.

these movements enables thumb opposition for the most delicate prehension as well as the most robust handling and grabbing objects. This joint is powered effectively by the 10 muscles surrounding it: flexor pollicis longus, extensor pollicis longus, extensor pollicis brevis, abductor pollicis longus, abductor pollicis brevis, flexor pollicis brevis, opponens pollicis, adductor pollicis caput obliquum, adductor pollicis caput transversum, and the first dorsal interosseous. These muscles are supplied by 3 major hand nerves (radial, median, and ulnar).

The stability of the unique double saddle joint is also aided by ligaments placed in a particular configuration. This is basic anatomic knowledge; it does not need to be repeated here. The forces exerted on this joint are more than 10 times the pinch force.[2] This unique joint makes it possible for the thumb to be very mobile under all kinds of applied loads while giving it adequate stability.

PATHOMECHANICS

It is still not entirely understood why this joint becomes arthritic mostly in women, and not more often in heavy manual workers. Moreover, the level of pain reported by patients does not always correlate with the degree of destruction seen radiologically. It is for this reason that the well-known Eaton classification of TMC1 joint osteoarthritis has very little clinical or practical value.

It is also our experience that the pinch strength of the thumb does not necessarily equate with the amount of destruction seen radiologically. The overwhelming complaint is pain, coupled with instability causing functional loss. Loss of dexterity and cosmetic abnormality, especially associated with a zig-zag collapse, are also reported.

In 1949, Gervis described treating these symptoms surgically and suggested trapezium excision.[3] In 1973, Eaton and Littler published on the treatment of osteoarthritis of this joint.[4] Later, Burton and Pellegrini in 1986 popularized the concept of ligamentous reconstruction and tendon interposition (LRTI).[5] Many surgeons have attempted to modify the LRTI operation. This has been followed by the development of numerous artificial prostheses to replace the TMC1 joint.

A recent count has shown that there are at least 40 stabilizing procedures (eg, ligament reconstructions) and more than 20 different prostheses. These facts alone indicate that many of these procedures are at best unreliable. Most of the proposed prostheses have been removed from the commercial market after only a few years because of their high failure rate.[6-8]

THE QUESTION AND CLINICAL GOALS

The question that needs to be answered is: what are the requirements for this unique joint to function optimally? I consider the minimum ideal requirements for a surgical procedure is offered are:

1. The operation has to be simple and easy to perform.
2. As osteoarthritis of TMC1 joint is very common, the surgery has to be affordable.
3. The operation should, if possible, not use any foreign material.
4. The procedure should be able to replicate much of the mechanical function of the TMC1 joint.
5. The operation should address the main symptoms, that is, pain and loss of function.
6. After the surgical reconstruction, the "new" joint has to be stable enough to allow reasonable pinch and grip function.
7. The surgical procedure has to offer a long-term predictable result for the patient and the surgeon.

A BALL-AND-SOCKET JOINT

From a biomechanical perspective, there can be no doubt that a ball-and-socket joint is inherently the most stable joint. It needs muscles to move it. The ligaments are therefore less important and contribute only a little to its stability and function mainly to limit its excursion (compare this to the hip joint when replaced by a prosthesis). The stability lies not in any ligament reconstruction, but in the shape of the new joint, that is, ball-and-socket.

The proximal articular shape of the trapezium bone is V-shaped and fits perfectly into the space created by the scaphoid head and the side of the trapezoid. The base of the thumb metacarpal (MC1) has a similar V-like shape (**Fig. 1**). Once the trapezium is removed, the 2 articular shapes fit quite nicely into each other in many cases, especially if the metacarpal (MC) is rotated a little into pronation, that is, the direction of opposition. As this is a "snug" fit (convex into concave shape), it can be regarded as a type of ball-and-socket joint.

ADVANTAGES OF A SIMPLE TRAPEZIUM EXCISION

By removing the whole of the trapezium, without inserting any autologous or foreign material, and allowing the MC base to sit into this new space, a sort of ball-and-socket joint is created. Any material or object inside the socket, would make the

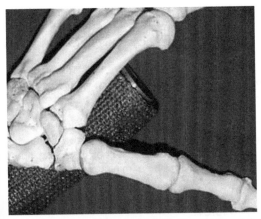

Fig. 1. The shape of the proximal joint surface of the first metacarpal matches the shape of the gap left when the trapezium is removed.

ball-and-socket concept unstable, as if in pole vaulting where the pole would be very unstable if the pole tip was planted in a vault box full of "stuff."

A simple and total removal of the trapezium has the following advantages[1]: The new ball-and-socket joint is reasonably stable in all directions.[2] As the original ligaments are left intact (the trapezium is removed), new ligaments need not be made, such as soft tissue reconstruction or stabilizing procedures as the ligaments reattach through scar tissue to the base of the MC.[3] The incision needed to perform this operation is small, no more than 15 to 20 mm long.[4] No foreign material or artificial material is inserted, reducing the risk of a foreign material reaction.[5] The operation is cheap because no expensive prosthesis is used.[6] The operating time is short, on average shorter than 30 minutes in my experience.[7] It follows logically from all the above that the complications should be much less than for larger/more complex procedures because there is less tissue damage.

Biomechanically, the narrow, adducted first web-space is relaxed because of the proximal "migration" of the MC. This releases the contracted tissues because of the longstanding abnormal position of the tissues surrounding the

thumb, allowing it to regain a more normal thumb position.

Because of this relaxation of the tight tissues, the hyperextension of the metacarpophalangeal (MCP) joint of the thumb is reduced and often does not require further treatment (**Fig. 2**). As the fulcrum of the thumb is moved slightly proximal, the improved lever arm allows the thumb to regain some of its power. As described earlier, the slightly rotated MC allows better opposition of the thumb.

SURGICAL TECHNIQUES

The surgical technique that we have consistently used is very straightforward and does not need special skills. In essence, it is removing the trapezium and associated degenerative tissue, inserting the first MC into the created socket, rotating it slightly into opposition, fixing the position with a single thin K-wire (0.5–0.6 mm), and closing the soft tissues (capsule, ligaments, and skin).

1. A bloodless field is made and maintained by an upper arm tourniquet. As WALANT has been popularized, this method may also be used.
2. A 15 to 20 mm incision is made on the radial side over the trapezium, taking care not to damage the branches of the radial nerve and the radial artery in the "snuff box." This incision lies longitudinally between the extensor pollicis longus and extensor pollicis brevis tendons.
3. The trapezium is fully removed piece-meal after releasing the ligaments from the trapezium. There is usually an osteophyte or a cartilaginous protrusion on the ulnar side at the base of the first MC, which must be removed to make it possible for the MC to subside into the new position (**Fig. 3**).
4. In cases of scaphotrapezoid joint arthritis, a 2 to 3 mm sliver of bone only is removed from the proximal part of the trapezoid. If this is not done, I consider that persistent residual pain may remain after surgery although the published research studies suggest this is not necessary (**Fig. 4**).

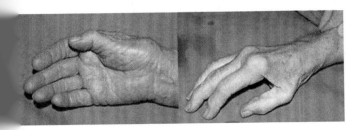

Fig. 2. The first web-space is restored, as well as the normal flexed position of the metacarpophalangeal joint after the trapeziectomy.

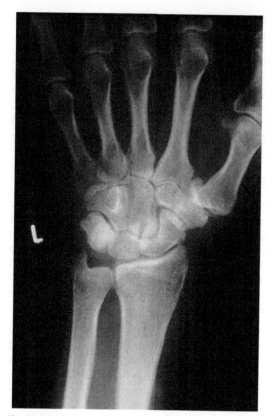

Fig. 3. It is essential that the osteophyte at the ulnar side at the base of the first metacarpal is removed. This may not always be seen on x-ray imaging because it may be cartilaginous, or still in an earlier phase of "development," that is, fibrous tissue.

5. The MC is now pushed into the hollow left by the removed trapezium, slightly rotated into opposition until the MC base settles into the "new" joint formed by the scaphoid head and the radial side of the trapezoid.
6. A single, thin K-wire (0.5–0.6 mm) is used to fix this position of abduction and opposition. The wire is drilled through the base of MC and into the trapezoid (or scaphoid head). It is cut short, leaving it protruding through the skin for 1 to 2 mm, or alternatively subcutaneously.
7. The exposed ligaments on the radial side including the capsule are sutured using only 1 or 2 absorbable 3/0 or 4/0 sutures. The skin is closed.
8. A forearm plaster-of-Paris slab is applied, which includes the thumb to hold it in the fixed position of abduction and opposition for 2 weeks.
9. At 2 weeks postoperatively, the K-wire is removed and a forearm cast is applied for another 3 weeks.

10. Mobilization can proceed immediately after the cast removal. Scar massage is encouraged to reduce adhesions. Physiotherapy is not typically required.

PATIENTS, RESULTS, AND COMPLICATIONS

The demographics of the patients treated from 1992 to 2014 (23 years) by the author are presented in **Table 1**. **Table 2** summarizes the results. The evaluations were recorded at varying times postoperatively, from a minimum of 2 years to 14 years postoperatively (**Fig. 5**).

DISCUSSION

Some authors have claimed that after simple trapezium excision-arthroplasty, the thumb ends up unacceptably short, that the pinch power is weak, that the first web-space becomes even narrower, that the thumb MCP joint remains in hyperextension, that the mobility of the thumb is compromised and that the thumb is unstable. I consider that these allegations are largely untrue and amount to perpetuated myths. The results presented earlier are based on a very large cohort over a relative long time and disproves these myths.

The slight overall shortening of the thumb of around 4 mm is usually of no significance. Only 3% of patients noted this slight shortening, for example, when holding a fork or writing with a pen. In this series, no patient reported this

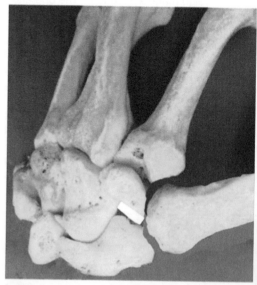

Fig. 4. When the scaphotrapezoid joint is degenerate, it is recommended to remove a 2-3 mm sliver from the proximal articular surface of the trapezoid to prevent chronic postoperative pain.

Table 1
Patient demographics

Patients seen	2183
Patients operated	1636 (75%)
Hands affected	3075
Both hands	1783 (58%)
One hand	1292 (42%)
Hands operated	2060 (67% of affected hands)
Sides	Left and right equal
Sex	
Female	86%
Male	14%
Age (22–86 y)	59 (mean)
Duration symptoms (1–30 y)	3.17 y (mean)
Main symptom	
Pain	93.7%
Weakness	3.7%
Other	2.6%
Pathology	
Osteoarthritis	94.8%
Trauma	3.7%
Rheumatoid arthritis	1.5%
Reoperations (referred): failed prostheses, failed arthrodesis, failed ligamentoplasties, etc.	44 Thumbs

shortening to be troublesome. Any surgery that eliminates pain and gives stability to the thumb should improve pinch power. In this series, we recorded an improvement of pinch power of 1.8 kg.

When the first MC subluxes (or even dislocates) secondary to TMC1 arthritis, the first web-space becomes compromised, that is, adducted. By excising the trapezium and moving the thumb complex a few millimeters proximally, the contracted tissue around the thumb is relaxed in part. This opens up the first web-space, and consequently improves the normal position of the thumb vis-à-vis the fingers. The first web-space opening improved by a mean of 27° in our series.

The compensating mechanism to "keep" the thumb out of the palm is hyperextension of the thumb MCP joint. The tight contracted first web-space that has been relaxed, helps to reduce the deforming forces on the thumb MCP joint leading to a more normal flexed position; in this series by a mean of 30°. In only 33 cases did we have to arthrodese the thumb MCP joint to provide MCP joint stability.

By virtue of the new "ball-and-socket-like joint," and the relaxation of the contracted tight tissue,

the thumb is once again able to oppose to the other digits and function more normally. We have never seen the so-called metacarpal-scaphoid impingement. We can only conclude that this might be a theoretic possibility but of no clinical importance.

Two surgical points need to be emphasized. First, the almost ever-present osteophyte, chondrophyte, or fibrophyte on the ulnar side at the base of the first MC bone must be sought and removed with a rongeur. This is essential to allow a snug seating in the scaphotrapezoid space. Secondly, we believe that if the scaphotrapezoid joint is also degenerated, that is, osteoarthritic, a small portion (about 2–3 mm) of the proximal part of the trapezoid must be removed although published studies have not shown this. In our experience, if this is not addressed, the patient will most likely still complain of pain after surgery, even if the operation was regarded as a "success."

Experience over 50 years of practicing medicine has taught me that the more complicated an answer to a clinical problem is, the further we move away from solving the issue at hand. Solving a painful base of the thumb osteoarthritic joint is a very good example of this principle. A glaringly

Table 2
Results

Pain: (pain was evaluated on a 5-point "Pain Severity Scale")		
0—No pain	48.9%	
1—Discomfort with certain activities	47.2%	
2—Some pain during daily activities	1.0%	
3—Intermittent spontaneous pain	2.0%	
4—Continuous pain	0.9%	
Pinch power: (Pinch meter) (overall improvement of 1.8 kg on preoperative values)	range 2–10 kg	3.6 kg
First web-space: (overall improvement of 27° on preoperative values)	range 60°–85°	75°
MCP joint: (position when pinching) flexion improved by 30°		
Stability: almost all patients (99%) reported noticeable improvement in thumb stability		
Thumb shortening: (only 3% of patients noticed any shortening without enquiry!)	range 2–6 mm	4 mm average
Opposition: (modified Kapanji 1–5)	5/5	98% of thumbs
Patient satisfaction: (VAS 1–10)		
Worse	1	1.3%
Same	3–4	2.9%
Satisfied	5–6	4.9%
Better	7–8	41.9%
Much better	9–10	49.0%
Complications:		
Subluxation of "new" joint (when pinching)	3 hands	
Stiffness (excessive scarring of skin incision)	6 hands	
Infection wound (diabetic patient)	4 hands	
Deep	0	
Instability of thumb when pinching (patients had hypermobile joints)	8 hands	
Scar tenderness	9 hands	
Cutaneous branches of the radial nerve injury	3 hands	
Residual pain (3 and 4/5)	60 hands	
Complex regional pain syndrome	5 hands (3 men, 2 women)	
Overall complication percentage:	4.8%	

simple solution has been made very complicated by very "clever" ideas such as innovative ligamentous reconstructions and prostheses.

The same aforementioned logical explanation applies to one of the most challenging procedures in hand surgery, namely pollicization. In the congenital deficient thumb, when a pollicization of the index finger is contemplated, it is not necessary to perform the complicated step to "make a trapezium" from the epiphysis of MC2. This making of a pseudotrapezium has always been part of various techniques described to "make a thumb." We have skipped this step in this operation, which not only reduced the operation time considerably but also reduced the manipulation of the delicate, small, and fragile tissue, and therefore reduced the potential for complications. The same reasoning and "myth-busting" arguments as pointed out earlier applies to a trapezium-less pollicization. The operative technique is even

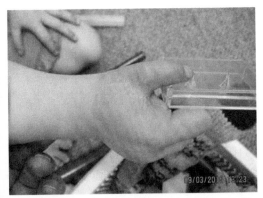

Fig. 5. Pollicization also does not need a trapezium. The pollicized finger is strong, stable, and looks cosmetically more like a thumb.

simpler than with the degenerative trapeziectomy. The MC of the intended finger to be pollicized is removed entirely, leaving a hollow where its base joined the carpus. The proximal phalanx is inserted into this gap, thus forming a ball-and-socket joint. The thumb is admittedly somewhat shorter, but looks cosmetically less like a finger, is inherently stable, can move in all the directions like a normal thumb, and is at least as powerful as a finger-like thumb[9] (**Fig. 6**).

SUMMARY

In the quest to restore what is broken in a body, surgeons have tried to simulate the "normal" and have tried to copy the intricate and sophisticated TMC1 joint of the human hand. This notion has been accepted as essential, that is, as an absolute, without question, and was transmitted from textbook to textbook, article to article, and teacher to student so many times that it has become

dogma without question. Most of us are therefore hesitant to even contemplate an alternative to such "fact set in stone."

This article challenges the idea that an artificial trapezium or reconstruction of new ligaments is necessary. Our large series followed over a long period shows very clearly that the results of a simple excision arthroplasty without any interposition or ligamentous "gymnastics" gives at least as good, if not better, results than any other proposed artificial procedure (see **Fig. 5**). We believe that any artificial prosthetic replacement of the trapezium is over operating and unnecessary.

CLINICS CARE POINTS

- When making the small 15 to 20 mm skin incision over the trapezium on the radial side of the wrist, take care not to damage the branches of the radial nerve or the radial artery.

- To protect the integrity of the ligaments, a subperiosteal release is done of the ligaments before the trapezium is removed piecemeal. These will attach to the base of the metacarpal during the healing phase.

- It is imperative to ensure complete removal of the trapezium.

- Always remove the osteophyte on the ulnar side at the base of the metacarpal. It may be cartilaginous or even only early excess fibrous tissue, which has not yet formed into an ossified osteophyte.

- When inserting the base of the metacarpal into the clean "socket," the snug fit will be better if the thumb is rotated a few degrees into the opposition position.

- If the trapezoid-scaphoid joint is degenerated, it is strongly advised to remove a small portion (2-3 mm) of the proximal articular joint surface of the trapezoid. This is an important step to prevent chronic pain or a "failed" operative procedure.

- Only 1 or 2 tight sutures are needed to close the capsule and incision in the surrounding ligamentous complex. This will add to the stability of the new base-of-thumb joint.

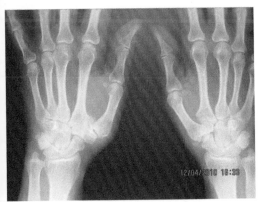

Fig. 6. Right hand postoperative radiographic image 14 years after a simple trapeziectomy for osteoarthritis of the first carpometacarpal joint. The joint space is maintained, and no impingement is seen. The left hand has not been operated upon.

REFERENCES

1. Gangopadhyay S, McKenna H, Burke FD, et al. Five to 18 year follow-up for treatment of trapeziometacarpal osteoarthritis: a prospective comparison of excision, tendon interposition, and ligament

reconstruction and tendon interposition. J Hand Surg Am 2012;37:411–7.

2. Brand PW. Clinical mechanics of the hand. C. V. Mosby; 1985. p. p50–4.

3. Gervis WH. Excision of the trapezium for osteoarthritis of the trapezio-metacarpal joint. J Bone Joint Surg Br 1949;31:537–9.

4. Eaton RG, Littler JW. Ligament reconstruction for the painful carpometacarpal joint. J Bone Joint Surg Am 1973;55:1655–66.

5. Burton RI, Pellegrini VD. Surgical management of basal joint arthritis of the thumb. Part II. Ligament reconstruction with tendon interposition arthroplasty. J Hand Surg Am 1986;11:324–32.

6. Huang K, Hollevoet N, Giddins G. Thumb carpometacarpal joint total arthroplasty: a systematic review. J Hand Surg Eur 2015;40:338–50.

7. Vermeulen GM, Slijper H, Feitz R, et al. Surgical management of primary thumb carpometacarpal osteoarthritis: a systematic review. J Hand Surg Am 2011;36:157–69.

8. Ganhewa AD, Wu R, Chae MP, et al. Failure rates of base of thumb arthritis surgery: a systematic review. J Hand Surg Am 2019;44:728–41.e10.

9. Mennen U. Pollicisation: The Myth about creating a pseudo-trapezium. J Hand Surg Asia-pacific 2018;23:302–30.

Dynamic Rather than Static Procedures in Correcting Claw Deformities Due to Ulnar Nerve Palsy

Brian W. Starr, MD*, Kevin C. Chung, MD, MS

KEYWORDS

• Ulnar nerve palsy • Clawing • Dynamic • Tendon transfers

KEY POINTS

- Surgical correction of ulnar nerve palsy and associated claw deformity remains a challenging undertaking with several viable treatment options.
- In the appropriately selected patient, both static and dynamic transfers can improve the claw deformity, namely through correction of metacarpophalangeal (MCP) joint hyperextension.
- However, comprehensive treatment can only be accomplished by effectively treating the underlying biomechanical disturbance that occurs because of loss of intrinsic function.
- Dynamic transfers aim to improve flexion synchrony, interphalangeal (IP) joint extension and overall grip strength—ambitious goals that static transfers are incapable of achieving.

Video content accompanies this article at http://www.hand.theclinics.com.

INTRODUCTION

Ulnar nerve palsy leads to a predictable and debilitating combination of functional disability and esthetic deformity. Progressive clawing of the ring and small fingers is arguably the most striking hallmark of ulnar nerve palsy; it is defined by resting hyperextension of the metacarpophalangeal (MCP) joints and flexion of the interphalangeal (IP) joints. Since the early 1900s, a multitude of surgical techniques have been proposed for the correction of claw deformity. Sterling Bunnell, Eduardo Zancolli, Daniel Riordan, Paul Brand, and other giants pioneered and continuously revised the approaches that form the basis of the most commonly used techniques today. Over the years, great minds have made reasonable arguments in support of both static and dynamic procedures. However, as our understanding of anatomy, biomechanics, and outcomes has evolved, so too has our approach to treatment. Unlike 1-dimensional static transfers, the dynamic transfers that we currently use in practice recreate some of the forces of deficient intrinsic musculature. These transfers aim to improve flexion synchrony, IP joint extension, and overall grip strength through the restoration of intrinsic biomechanics. In critically evaluating the fundamental basis and efficacy of these techniques, we contend that dynamic procedures are undoubtedly superior to their static counterparts.

PATHOPHYSIOLOGY AND BIOMECHANICS

The interosseous muscles are predominantly responsible for both MCP joint flexion and IP joint extension in the fingers. In the case of ulnar nerve palsy, loss of the ulnar-innervated interossei and

Section of Plastic Surgery, The University of Michigan Health System, 1500 East Medical Center Drive, 2130 Taubman Center, SPC 5340, Ann Arbor, MI 48109-5340, USA

* Corresponding author.

E-mail address: starrbri@med.umich.edu

Hand Clin 38 (2022) 313–319
https://doi.org/10.1016/j.hcl.2022.02.008
0749-0712/22/© 2022 Elsevier Inc. All rights reserved.

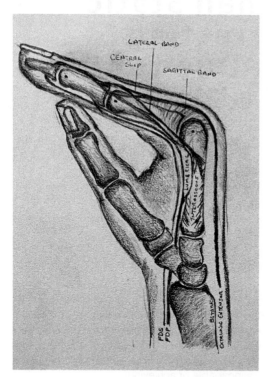

Fig. 1. Diagram of intrinsic musculature. Under normal circumstances, interossei and lumbricals exert a flexion force at the MCP joint and an extension force at the IP joints.

lumbrical muscles leads to predictable intrinsic minus "claw" deformity and deterioration of cohesive hand function. The harmonious interplay between intrinsic and extrinsic forces is essential to maintain both fine and gross motor skills, as well as the basic resting posture of the hand. Under normal circumstances, the interosseous musculotendinous unit transmits force volar to the axis of rotation of the MCP joints and dorsal to the axis of rotation of the IP joints (**Fig. 1**). In the case of ulnar nerve palsy, devoid of interossei-led MP joint flexion and IP joint extension, the balance between intrinsic and extrinsic forces is devastated.

Loss of the ulnar-nerve–innervated lumbrical muscles to the ring and small fingers exacerbates the claw deformity and the loss of flexion-extension synchrony. Biomechanical studies indicate that the primary motor function of the lumbrical muscles is to assist in IP joint extension, albeit to a lesser extent than the interossei.[1] Based on the biomechanical work of Buford and colleagues, the lumbricals have been shown to be responsible for just 2% of the total moment arm at the MCP joint flexion. By comparison, the interossei account for 22% of the total flexion moment at the MCP joint.[2] Their limited contribution can be partly

because their cross-sectional area and muscle mass is the smallest in the upper extremity. Although weak, the lumbricals are dense in muscle fibrils. In combination with its unique flexor origin and extensor insertion, it is theorized that the lumbrical muscles primarily serve sensory and proprioceptive feedback to help optimize smooth movements of the digits. Despite their limited work potential, the median-nerve–innervated index and long finger lumbricals play a noticeable role in preventing the progression of claw deformity in these digits.

At rest, in the absence of intrinsic muscle tone, the sagittal bands are oriented parallel to the central slip over the proximal interphalangeal (PIP) joint. The extensor mechanism, now dependent solely on the extrinsic extensor tendon and central slip, transmits its force to the proximal phalanx, thus hyperextending the MCP joint. With the MCP joint in hyperextension, the central slip reaches the limit of its excursion earlier in the ranges of movement and is unable to exert more than limited extension force at the PIP joint. The deformity is compounded by the unopposed action of the extrinsic finger flexor tendons, which are placed on stretch by MCP joint hyperextension and subsequently drive the IP joints into flexion. The claw deformity, is more pronounced in "low" ulnar nerve injuries, due to intact and unopposed flexor digitorum profundus forces that exacerbate IP joint flexion (**Fig. 2**).

Beyond the resting claw deformity that develops, active function is also severely impaired. Ordinarily, MCP and IP joint flexion occur simultaneously and in tandem. However, with loss of the intrinsics, the hand loses its primary MCP joint flexor. Relying solely on the extrinsic flexors, MCP joint flexion only occurs after sequential distal interphalangeal and PIP joint flexion. From a practical standpoint, this makes grasping large objects nearly impossible. Grip contact area decreases up to 90% with the tips of the fingers curled to the metacarpal heads.[3] Grip strength is also dramatically reduced by up to 75% with the loss of intrinsic function.[4–6]

The preceding summary of the delicate biomechanics at the heart of the disability and deformity of ulnar nerve palsy points to a clear solution: dynamic intrinsic reconstruction. Claw deformity and the loss of grip strength, dexterity, and overall function are inseparably intertwined with the state of the intrinsic musculature. Static procedures fail to address the fundamental problem with loss of intrinsic forces and instead settle for treating one part of the larger problem. Although there is no perfect solution to restore lost intrinsic function, dynamic procedures can offer a fine imitator.

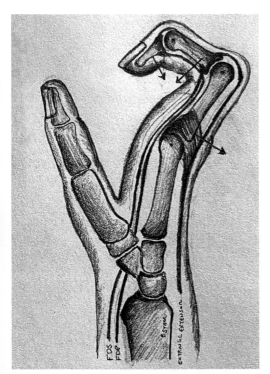

Fig. 2. Clawing of the ring and small fingers seen in a patient with low ulnar nerve palsy. Denervated intrinsic muscles removed. Arrows demonstrate force vector exerted by extrinsic muscles relative to the joints.

SURGICAL TECHNIQUES
Static Procedures

The singular, direct aim of static procedures is to correct MCP joint hyperextension. In placing the MCP joints in neutral or in slight flexion, these procedures aim to augment extrinsic extensor excursion and enhance the extension force directed to the IP joints through the central slip. Static procedures may correct clawing; however, they fail to improve grip strength or flexion synchrony. Static techniques are less versatile and more limited in their application than dynamic techniques. In particular, static procedures are contraindicated in patients with a negative Bouvier test. In this test, MP joint extension is blocked by the examiner, and active IP joint extension is assessed. A positive test result is achieved if the patient is able to actively extend at the PIP joint, indicating an intact central slip. We are skeptical of tenodesis procedures for which medical illustrations substantially outnumber clinical photos—not to mention published results. Arthrodesis of the finger MCP joints remains a last-resort, salvage operation reserved for those with high combined ulnar nerve palsies for which limited donor tendons

are available for the dynamic transfer; fusion should not be applied routinely for functional reconstruction. For these reasons, we cannot advocate static tenodesis or arthrodesis procedures and will not review them in this text.

Volar Plate Capsulodesis

Probably the most frequently performed static procedure, volar plate capsulodesis at the MCP joint was originally developed by Zancolli in 1954. The idea for the technique reportedly stemmed from Zancolli's observing the absence of clawing in patients with burns, contractures, MCP joint adhesions, congenital volar plate shortening, and other conditions that effectively prevented MCP joint hyperextension.[7,8] The technique itself applies an approach akin to a trigger finger release, with a volar incision over the A1 pulley of the affected digit. The A1 pulley is divided and the flexor tendons are retracted laterally to expose the MCP joint volar plate. The volar plate is then detached from the metacarpal neck, as a distally based flap, and advanced proximally. Proximal advancement tension should be set sufficiently taut to ensure adequate MCP joint flexion and subsequent IP joint extension. The volar plate is either imbricated with nonabsorbable sutures proximally, or, alternatively can be reinserted to the metacarpal itself through bone tunnels and suture anchors.[7] The procedure is alluring, in part, because of its apparent simplicity. However, the simplicity is a mirage, because full exposure of the volar plate and the metacarpal bone in the depth of the palmar hand is not possible unless an unacceptably long incision is made for each digit. Beyond an inherent failure to overcome the deficiency in intrinsic forces, capsulodesis procedures are flawed in that they are prone to attenuation, stretching, and recurrence of MCP joint hyperextension over time.

Dynamic Procedures

From a biomechanical standpoint, dynamic procedures offer clear advantages over static procedures. By adding a motor that mirrors the lost intrinsic musculature, dynamic procedures attempt to overcome the most essential defect in the intrinsic minus hand. In doing so, dynamic procedures can overcome the claw deformity, the weakened grip, and flexion asynchrony.

Wrist Motor Transfers

Brand transfer
The "Brand" extensor carpi radialis brevis (ECRB) transfer was initially described by Littler in 1949, and later revised and popularized by Brand in

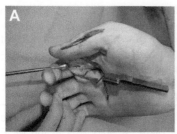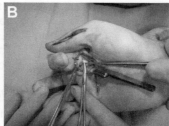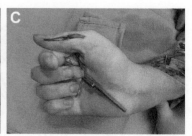

Fig. 3. Zancolli Lasso procedure. (*A*) Flexor tendon sheath (*) identified and a window is made in the distal A2 pulley (). (*B*) FDS tendon (+) transected distally at its insertion. (*C*) FDS tendon (+) looped proximally over the A1 pulley (−) and sutured on itself.

1992.[9] The technique uses the ECRB musculotendoninous complex as a motor, augmented with a tendon graft, to reestablish intrinsic function. Through a dorsal incision over the third metacarpal, the ECRB tendon is identified and divided at its insertion on the third metacarpal base. A tendon graft, typically palmaris longus, is harvested and woven into the distal end of the ECRB tendon. The distal end of the tendon graft is divided into 2 or 4 slips, depending on the number of recipient digits selected. The radial lateral bands are identified through separate midlateral incisions over the proximal phalanges. The slips of graft are then tunneled dorsal-to-volar and through the lumbrical canals before being woven into the radial lateral bands. It is critical to ensure that the transferred tendon is passed volar to the deep transverse intermetacarpal ligament before redirecting the transfer dorsally to its distal insertion. This new course will provide a flexion vector at the MP joint while simultaneously adding an extension force on the IP joints. Variations in insertion sites can have a dramatic impact on the role of the transfer and overall restoration of function. When there is a positive Bouvier test (ie, the existing extensor mechanism is capable of extending the IP joints), the transferred tendon can be secured to the A1 or A2 pulley, or inserted into a bone tunnel. Conversely, if the extensor mechanism is incompetent, as demonstrated by a negative Bouvier test, then the tendon transfer must be inserted into the lateral band to restore IP joint extension.

FDS transfers: Zancolli lasso transfer

Although the Zancolli lasso procedure is, by definition, a dynamic procedure because a tendon is used, it does not address the intrinsic deficit and therefore shares some of the shortcomings of static procedures. By releasing and rerouting the FDS tendon around the A1 pulley and onto itself, the lasso procedure creates a "dynamic tether" that aims to correct MCP joint hyperextension

(**Fig. 3**).[8] The procedure does not recreate intrinsic force and therefore fails to augment IP joint extension or grip strength.[10]

Authors' Preferred Technique: Modified Stiles-Bunnell Transfer

The theoretic disadvantage of dynamic tendon transfers is the perception that they are "more complex," technically and for patient rehabilitation. In our practice, we have consistently achieved reasonable correction of claw deformity and improvement in tendon synchrony and grip strength with a modified Stiles-Bunnell transfer. As described in Littler's modification of the classic technique, we use one FDS tendon to restore intrinsic force to the ring and small fingers.[11] We preferentially select the FDS to the long finger as our donor motor, provided that the innervation of the long finger FDS from the median nerve is intact.

Preoperatively, the incision sites are marked for the FDS donor tendon harvest and for the insertion of the transfer into the radial lateral bands (**Fig. 4**A). Through a volar, Brunauer incision over the donor finger, the FDS tendon is identified just distal to its decussation at the Camper chiasm (**Fig. 4**B). A window is made in the A3 pulley and the FDS tendon is divided at its insertion over the middle of the middle phalanx (**Fig. 4**C). The FDS tendon is then retracted into the palm and dissected free of surrounding synovial attachments (**Fig. 4**D). To obtain adequate length of the individual FDS donor slips, it is necessary to split the FDS tendon several additional centimeters, proximal to its natural decussation (**Fig. 4**E). Midlateral incisions are then made over the radial aspect of the ring and small fingers. Blunt dissection identifies the lateral bands (**Fig. 4**F). A curved hemostat is then used to develop the subcutaneous tunnel from the midlateral incisions distally, through the lumbrical canal, to the FDS donor tendon in the palm. The critical point here is to

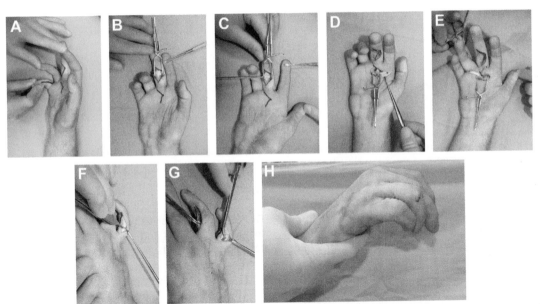

Fig. 4. Author's preferred technique—modified Stiles-Bunnell transfer. (*A*) Incisions marked. (*B*) FDS tendon (+) identified at its insertion. (*C*) FDS tendon divided. (*D*) FDS tendon (+) retrieved through proximal incision. (*E*) Splitting of FDS slips (+). (*F*) Radial lateral band () identified. (*G*) FDS slips (+) woven into radial lateral band (). (*H*) Resting posture, intraoperatively, following transfer.

ensure that the tunnel, starting from the relatively dorsal lateral band, is developed *volar* to the deep metacarpal ligament. The FDS slips are retrieved in the palm and passed through the tunnel to their distal insertion sites. A small incision is made in the midline of the radial lateral band and the FDS tendon is woven through and sutured on itself (**Fig. 4**G). The tension is set slightly tighter than a normal resting cascade—approximately 60 to 70 degrees of flexion at the MCP joint, with the IP joints fully extended and the wrist in slight extension—to ensure good flexion and extension on tenodesis testing (**Fig. 4**H). The transfer is secured with two or three 3-0 nonabsorbable Ethibond horizontal mattress sutures. The patient is immobilized in an intrinsic plus volar splint for 4 weeks postoperatively. At 4 weeks postoperatively, the patient is transitioned to a dorsal-blocking removable splint and begins gentle active range of motion exercises. At 8 weeks postoperatively, the splint is discontinued, and activity restrictions are lifted.

OUTCOMES

In 1969, Brown performed a meticulous review of 44 patients treated with static procedures composed of 109 volar plate capsulodeses. At a mean of 2 years postoperatively, only 21 of 44 patients (48%) demonstrated sustained improvement in positioning and clawing, with improved grasp.[12]

In a retrospective review of 44 patients, Ozkan and colleagues compared the 3, previously discussed dynamic transfer techniques; the modified Stiles Bunnell transfer, the Zancolli lasso transfer, and the Brand transfer.[13] At a mean of 48 months postoperatively, each dynamic transfer was effective in restoring grip strength, with the modified Stiles Bunnell, FDS transfer, being the most effective transfer in correcting clawing. In a review of 127 hands treated with FDS transfer for intrinsic reconstruction, Brandsma and colleagues reported excellent results in 21% and "good" results in 57%, with swan-neck deformity affecting 15% of donor digits at a mean postoperative follow-up of 6.5 years.[14] Similarly, we have seen good-to-excellent results in most of our patients treated with this technique. **Fig. 5**A–C and Video 1 demonstrate a typical postoperative result at 3 months follow-up. In Ozkan's series, the authors reported a postoperative complication of swan-neck deformity that occurred in 7 recipient digits treated with the modified Stiles Bunnell transfer.[13] The risk of swan-neck deformity is a well-documented complication in cases of FDS transfer, and can occur to donor and recipient digits. This deformity does not occur frequently, because the claw hand typically has contracted PIP joint, and even with a tight repair over the lateral band, the PIP joint should maintain some residual flexion contracture.

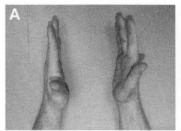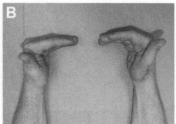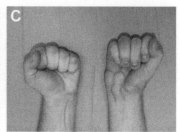

Fig. 5. (*A–C*) Postoperative result following modified Stiles-Bunnell transfer at 3-months follow-up.

SUMMARY

The hallmarks of ulnar nerve palsy include deforming intrinsic minus posturing and disabling weakness affecting pinch and grip strength, dexterity, and fine motor control. Before undertaking surgical correction, the hand surgeon must have a firm understanding of the underlying intrinsic and extrinsic anatomy, and biomechanical principles. Although they are effective in correcting claw deformity in select patients, static procedures oversimplify the problem and fail to address disturbances in strength and asynchrony distal to the MCP joints. Dynamic transfers offer a comprehensive approach and aim to improve flexion synchrony, IP joint extension, and overall grip strength through the restoration of intrinsic biomechanics.

CLINICS CARE POINTS

- In patients presenting with ulnar nerve palsy, both static and dynamic procedures can potentially correct clawing by addressing deforming forces about the MCP joint.
- Static procedures are only effective in correcting clawing in patients with a positive Bouvier test preoperatively, and will not improve flexion synchrony, IP joint extension, or grip strength.
- By mimicking the force and direction of pull of the lost intrinsic musculature, dynamic transfers correct claw deformity and improve flexion synchrony, IP joint extension, and grip strength.
- Our preferred dynamic tendon transfer is the modified Stiles-Bunnell (FDS) transfer. Care must be taken to ensure the FDS tendon is passed volar to the deep metacarpal ligament before being inserted dorsally into the radial lateral band.

DISCLOSURE

Dr K.C. Chung receives funding from the National Institutes of Health and book royalties from Wolters Kluwer and Elsevier. He is a consultant for Axogen.

SUPPLEMENTARY DATA

Supplementary data related to this article can be found online at .https://doi.org/10.1016/j.hcl.2022.02.008.

REFERENCES

1. Wang K, McGlinn EP, Chung KC. A biomechanical and evolutionary perspective on the function of the lumbrical muscle. J Hand Surg Am 2014;39:149–55.
2. Buford WL Jr, Koh S, Andersen CR, et al. Analysis of intrinsic-extrinsic muscle function through interactive 3-dimensional kinematic simulation and cadaver studies. J Hand Surg Am 2005;30:1267–75.
3. Brand PW, Hunter JM, Schneider LH, et al. Tendon surgery in the hand. St. Louis, MO: CV Mosby; 1987. p. 439–53.
4. Smith RJ. Tendon transfers of the hand and forearm. First Edition ed. Boston, Brown: Little; 1987.
5. Goldfarb CA, Stern PJ. Low ulnar nerve palsy. J Am Soc Surg Hand 2003;3:14–26.
6. Kozin SH, Porter S, Clark P, et al. The contribution of the intrinsic muscles to grip and pinch strength. J Hand Surg Am 1999;24:64–72.
7. Sapienza A, Green S, et al. Correction of the claw hand. Hand Clin 2012;28:53–66.
8. Zancolli EA. Claw hand caused by paralysis of the intrinsic muscles. A simple surgical procedure for its correction. J Bone Joint Surg Am 1957;1076–80.
9. Brandsma JW, Brand PW. Claw-finger correction. considerations in choice of technique. J Hand Surg Br 1992;17:615–21.
10. Hastings H 2nd, McCollam SM. Flexor digitorum superficialis lasso tendon transfer in isolated ulnar nerve palsy: A functional evaluation. J Hand Surg Am 1994;19:275–80.

11. Littler JW. Tendon transfers and arthrodeses in combined median and ulnar nerve paralysis. J Bone Joint Surg Am 1949;31:225–34.

12. Brown PW. Zancolli capsulorrhaphy for ulnar claw hand. appraisal of forty-four cases. J Bone Joint Surg Am 1970;52:868–77.

13. Ozkan T, Ozer K, Gülgönen A. Three tendon transfer methods in reconstruction of ulnar nerve palsy. J Hand Surg Am 2003;28:35–43.

14. Brandsma JW, Ottenhoff-de Jonge MW. Flexor digitorum superficialis tendon transfer for intrinsic replacement: Long-term results and the effect on donor fingers. J Hand Surg Br 1992;17:625–8.

Some Misconceptions in the Treatment of Cubital Tunnel Syndrome, Radial Tunnel Syndrome, and Median Nerve Compression in the Forearm

Jin Bo Tang, MD

KEYWORDS

- Ulnar nerve • Radial nerve • Median nerve • Compression • Cubital tunnel syndrome
- Radial tunnel syndrome • Lacertus syndrome • FDS-Pronator syndrome

KEY POINTS

- Struthers' ligament extremely rarely causes ulnar neuropathy and it does not occur together with cubital tunnel syndrome. Exploration of this ligament is not suggested if definitive compression is found at cubital tunnel release. Compression to the ulnar nerve proximal to the elbow can be detected with ultrasound; the release should be directed to the site proximal to the elbow.
- Lacertus syndrome and flexor superficialis-pronator syndrome are different entities and can be diagnosed separately. Surgical release can be through a small incision. A lengthy incision to explore and release all possible sites of compression is unnecessary.
- Acronyms for compression to radial nerve in proximal forearm can be simplified to be one, that is, radial tunnel syndrome; this includes a mild type (classical radial tunnel syndrome) and a severe type (posterior interosseous nerve (PIN) compression).

INTRODUCTION

I choose to write on this topic because my treatment of these patients has changed over the decades, from closely following recommendations in textbooks to my current approach. Some of these disorders are very uncommon so it took me many years to revise my treatment methods. In this article, I summarize my recommended approaches and discuss what should be revised in the published texts.

CUBITAL TUNNEL SYNDROME
Definitions

Cubital tunnel syndrome is used interchangeably with ulnar nerve compression in the elbow region.

Clinically, cubital tunnel syndrome should indicate the compression of ulnar nerve in the cubital tunnel area, which is at the elbow joint level. This does not include the area proximal to the elbow; latter should be considered separately.

By this definition, the structures of the Osborne's ligament, the fascia between 2 heads of flexor carpi ulnaris (FCU), and any condensed fibrotic tissues around the ulnar nerve can cause cubital tunnel syndrome (**Figs. 1** and **2**). Secondary compression can occur from elbow arthritis and rarely local tumors.

The Osborne's ligament only covers a part of the cubital tunnel.[1–4] The cubital tunnel locates in the area posterior to the medial epicondyle from the site of fascia between 2 heads of the FCU tendon

Department of Hand Surgery, Affiliated Hospital of Nantong University, Nantong, Jiangsu, China
E-mail address: jinbotang@yahoo.com

Hand Clin 38 (2022) 321–328
https://doi.org/10.1016/j.hcl.2022.02.003
0749-0712/22/© 2022 Elsevier Inc. All rights reserved.

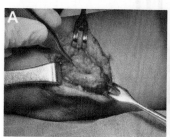 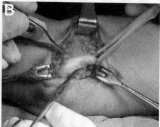

Fig. 1. (*A*) Fibrotic tissue surrounding the ulnar nerve causing compression. (*B*) After excision of the fibrotic compressive tissues around the nerve. (*Courtesy of Jin Bo Tang, MD, Jiangsu, China*).

to the upper margin of the medial epicondyle (**Figs. 3** and **4**). This ligament is the ligamentous tissue connecting the olecranon and the medial epicondyle. This ligament has varying incidence (77-100%) and can be thin or thick, and it varies individually in width and configuration as well as exact location.[1–4] The Osborne's ligament usually covers the distal or/and middle part of the tunnel if present (see **Fig. 3**).

In the patients with cubital tunnel syndrome, condensed fibrotic tissues around the ulnar nerve often form a constrictive sleeve around the nerve or in some cases a dense layer of fibrotic tissue directly covering the ulnar nerve at the elbow region, likely because of repetitive elbow motion or over use. I consider *fibrotic tissues* that directly compress the ulnar nerve, rather than the Osborne's ligament. These fibrotic tissues are not often mentioned in textbooks, but I consider these tissues between the nerve and the Osborne's ligament initiate the compression to the nerve; all the fibrotic tissues have to be excised or released after releasing the Osborne's ligament.

In patients without an apparent Osborne's ligament, cubital tunnel syndrome still occurs, due to

fibrotic tissues around the ulnar nerve; I consider the presence of the Osborne's ligament only makes the compression more severe.

The Sites not Needing Routine Attention or Release

Based on the literature, the incidence of compression to the ulnar nerve by the *Struthers'* ligament is extremely rare (**Fig. 5**). In the published English literature only 1 case has been reported.[5] Surveys of senior surgeons typically report never having seen a case.[6] I have never seen and neither have the 15 other colleagues in my department.

It should be also stressed that ulnar nerve compression by this ligament in that reported case did not occur with the cubital tunnel compression, and no report of simultaneous occurrence of compression at 2 sites.[5,6] Therefore, when a surgeon has completed releasing constriction in the cubital tunnel, there is no reason to explore the area of the *Struthers'* ligament.

Given the rarity of ulnar nerve compression caused by the ligament of Struthers, I recommend it should not be explored routinely at ulnar nerve

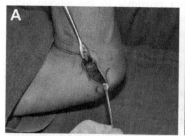 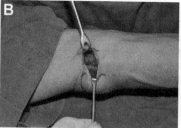 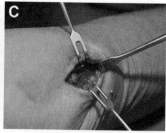

Fig. 2. The release of compressive, fibrotic tissue over the ulnar nerve in a mild case with mini-incision of 3 cm: (*A*) compression by a layer of fibrotic tissue proximally (partially excised already), (*B*) The thin fibrotic tissue layer in the middle part of the cubital tunnel, and (*C*) Distally the thin fibrotic tissue also noted, which should also be released. The compressive tissue with fibrosis is usually found in the entire cubital tunnel posterior to the ulnar groove as seen in this mild case. The Osborne's ligament covers only the middle part of the tunnel. Release of only this ligament would not decompress the ulnar nerve. It is a key to release any compressive (usually fibrotic) tissues over the ulnar nerve in the area of the cubital tunnel. It is the fibrotic compressive tissues superficial or around the ulnar nerve in the entire cubital tunnel (deeper to Osborne's ligament) that cause the compression. In other words, Osborne's ligament likely not initiate the compression at all. The fibrotic compressive tissue is the reason for ulnar neuropathy in the elbow area.

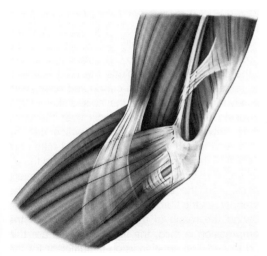

Fig. 3. The Osborne's ligament. Its width varies individually. Some investigators describe it as a narrower structure covering only the distal part of the area. (*Courtesy of* Julia Ruston, MBBS, London, UK).

decompression and its rarity should be emphasized more clearly in the textbooks.

In the few reported cases, patients were found to present with pain and tenderness about 10 cm proximal to the cubital tunnel with motor and sensory disturbance of ulnar nerve area distally. The ulnar nerve was compressed by the muscles or fibrous bands; only one caused by the Struthers' ligament.5 The chance of encountering such cases is very rare. If encountered, radiographs should be performed to see whether there is a bony spur, or an ultrasound to assess for ulnar nerve compression in the distal arm.

The term "arcade of Struthers" was created by Kane and colleagues.[7,8] They described that the

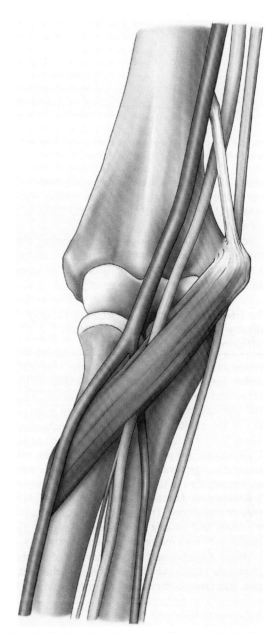

Fig. 5. The Struthers' ligament. (*Courtesy of* Julia Ruston, MBBS, London, UK)

internal brachial ligament "forms an arcade for passage of the ulnar nerve" and that it "appears to be a tendinous attachment of part of the medial head of the triceps in the lower third of the humerus." This arcade was found in 14 of 20 (70%) arms dissected.[7] They described it as having a roof 2 cm wide and reinforced by superficial fibers of the medial head of the triceps and thickening of the deep investing fascia of the arm. Its anterior border is the thickened medial intermuscular septum and its lateral aspect is the deep muscular fibers of the medial head of the triceps. Kane and

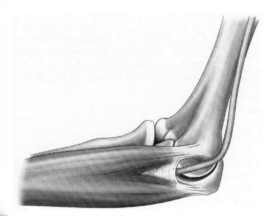

Fig. 4. The 2 heads of the FCU tendon and their relation to the ulnar nerve. (*Courtesy of* Julia Ruston, MBBS, London, UK)

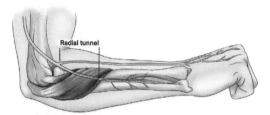

Fig. 6. The boundaries of the radial tunnel. (*Courtesy of* Julia Ruston, MBBS, London, UK)

colleagues[7] described it as having a close relationship to the ulnar nerve, rather than finding compressing it. This term is different from *Struthers'* ligament.

Wehrli and Oberlin suggested canceling this term.[9] Considering the rarity of these structures as a cause of ulnar nerve compression,[10-12] I agree this term should no longer be used.

The Sites and Structures to Release During Surgery and a Small Incision is Often Sufficient

In patients with cubital tunnel syndrome, I carefully localize the site of pain and tenderness at the elbow, and perform surgical release at the sites of tenderness, commonly within 4 to 5 cm in the region of the cubital tunnel. A surgical incision of around 3 to 4 cm is usually sufficient. Only 3 types of structures are released during surgery: (1) Osborne's ligament; it is often mixed with condensed, fibrotic tissue around the ulnar nerve. (2) Condensed fibrotic tissue around the ulnar nerve at the elbow. This kind of tissue presents very often, and usually very dense, except in the patients with very mild compression. I often have to release a condensed layer or sheath of fibrotic tissue over or around the ulnar nerve if the ulnar nerve has been compressed for a long time. (3)

The more distally located fascia between the 2 heads of the FCU tendon. The fascia can be compressive, but is usually not as dense as the fibrotic tissues deeper into Osborne's ligament or in the cubital tunnel. I include the FCU fascia in the release as this can be conducted easily with slightly forceful traction on the incised skin distally exposing the thin layer of fascia over the ulnar nerve between muscle bundles, which can be cut over a length of about 1 to 2 cm. I take care to confirm the dense fibrotic tissues around the ulnar nerve is excised completely in rather severe cases, and the skin incision may need to be extended as the fibrotic tissues sometimes extend beyond the reach of the original incision. If the compression is mild, the fibrotic tissues are thin and limited, the small incision is sufficient for the release. The complete decompression of the ulnar nerve can be confirmed by direct visualization.

I do not release or explore beyond these structures, although I do take care to exclude any space-occupying lesions (such as ganglion or other tumors) in this area.

If ulnar nerve compression is secondary to severe elbow arthritis, I recommend the treatment of arthritis with bony procedures first and the ulnar nerve should be transposed anteriorly. The patients with severe elbow arthritis are usually considered different from patients without arthritis.

RADIAL TUNNEL SYNDROME

Confusing acronyms are used to describe radial nerve compression.[13-22] In my experience there are two distinct presentations. I consider we can simplify the acronyms under only one term "*radial tunnel syndrome*" (**Figs. 6** and **7**). There is a mild type (with pain and sometimes sensory disturbance) and a severe type (with motor dysfunction

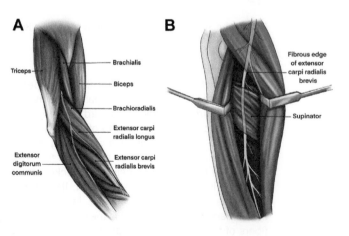

Fig. 7. Location of the radial tunnel and related structures around the radial nerve. (*A*) lateral view. (*B*) dorsal view. (*Courtesy of* Julia Ruston, MBBS, London, UK)

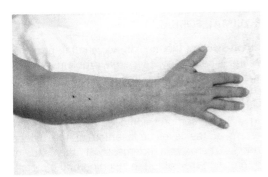

Fig. 8. Site of tenderness of the patient with radial tunnel syndrome is between 2 dots, which is the site of incision for exploration and release. This patient has incision between 2 dots, over the site of tenderness. (*Courtesy of* Jin Bo Tang, MD, Jiangsu, China)

with weakness of the muscles innervated by the posterior interosseous nerve (PIN). These 2 presentations cover what are traditionally considered 2 different disorders, that is, radial tunnel syndrome and PIN compression. I have detailed why I propose referring to them both as radial tunnel syndrome in a recent article.[23]

Surgical Treatment: Under One Term with Similar Approaches

I use a small incision (about 3–5 cm), targeting at the site of tenderness or sites of abnormal findings in preoperative ultrasound or MRI scans (**Fig. 8**). Scans help detect or exclude any space-occupying lesions or constriction of the radial nerve before surgery. I consider the location of the local tenderness is of the utmost importance in diagnosis. In the milder type of radial tunnel syndrome, tenderness can usually be localized precisely, about 4 to 5 cm distal to the lateral epicondyle over the route of the PIN. Though, the PIN is deep under the muscle, or travels between muscles, the site of tenderness is distinctive; in particular, it is distal to the lateral epicondylar tenderness seen in patients with tennis elbow.

Via a 3 to 5 cm incision centered over the site of tenderness, the radial nerve can be exposed,

either accessing between the ECRB and brachioradialis muscle bellies, or more commonly between the ECRB-extensor digitorum communis (EDC) interval, the PIN can be found. With skin retraction a reasonable length of the PIN can be explored (**Fig. 9**). The site of the ECRB crossing the PIN, the leash of Henry, and the arcade of Frohse can be explored, and usually released. Nerve compression may not be seen clearly because compression in most of these patients is mild. It is best to release these sites in the region that surgical incision can expose, and remove any possible (not confirmative) compressive tissues away from the PIN. The release often includs cut the arcade of Frohse as this structure often causes problems. If preoperative scans show a tumor or constrictive band around the PIN, the tumor or band should be explored and addressed. In the patients with a definitive cause of compression such as a tumor or a constricting band, I wound also explore the sites of other nearby possible compression sites such as arcade of Frohse and the site of ECRB crossing the PIN, which is often in the operating field, because these sites easily compress the PIN with the presence of scar or chronic inflammatory or fibrotic tissues; therefore, these sites need to be checked and cleaned even a tumor is removed. I do not explore all the possible sites of compression as it is not reasonable. A large incision is needed for extensive exploration to all possible compression sites, which is usually unnecessary.

I have not encountered a case of radial nerve compression secondary to an arthritic elbow joint, and I assume this can be diagnosed through plain X-ray films and clinical findings of the radial nerve compression and the exploration and surgical release should be confined to the site of compression in the elbow joint, and usually a surgery through an anterior approach, and other sites of compression should not be explored, as the etiology of the compression already known. Radial nerve compression by the abnormal elbow joint is different from radial nerve compression by muscles and tendinous tissues.

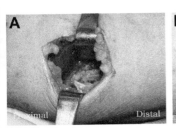
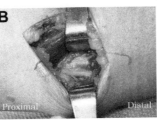

Fig. 9. The same patient of **Fig. 8** and the radial nerve was exposed through the incision. The incision exposed the radial nerve longer than the length of incision, because the skin incision can be pulled proximally (*A*) and distally (*B*) to access a wider scope of tissues. (*Courtesy of* Jin Bo Tang, MD, Jiangsu, China)

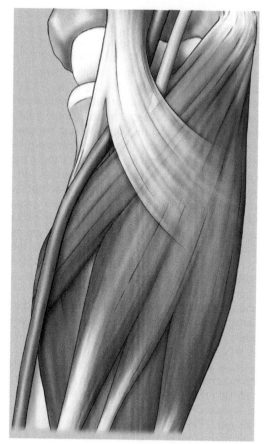

Fig. 10. Lacertus fibrosus and its relation with the median nerve. (*Courtesy of* Julia Ruston, MBBS, London, UK)

MEDIAN NERVE COMPRESSION IN THE PROXIMAL FOREARM

Compression of the median nerve in the proximal forearm is caused by 2 separate problems: (1) *lacertus syndrome*: this is compression of the median nerve by the aponeurosis of biceps tendons, that is, the bicipital aponeurosis or lacertus fibrosus (**Fig. 10**). The compression occurs in the proximal forearm at the level of insertion of the biceps tendon. There is tenderness at the site of compression medial to the insertion of the biceps tendon. A very small incision of 2 cm is sufficient to release the cause, the lacertus fibrosus.[24–26] (2) *FDS-pronator syndrome*: this is compression of the median nerve by either the FDS or pronator muscles (**Fig. 11**).[26,27] This occurs slightly more distal than the lacertus syndrome where the median nerve passes between the heads of the FDS and pronator muscles. Release of part of the pronator muscle is usually necessary as well as part of the tendinous arch of the origin of the FDS. Differentiating between the origin of the FDS and deep part of the pronator is not easy during surgery. In doubt, any tight muscle fibers or bands should be released. I have found in several patients the tendinous bands tensioned over the median nerve. I used my index fingertip to check the tension of the muscles or tendinous structures over the median nerve. My surgical incision for exploring median nerve compression in the FDS-pronator syndrome is usually not large (4–5 cm). I have not found any patients with definite compression by the FDS-pronator also having compression at the site of the lacertus fibrosus, but if the lacertus fibrosus can be seen proximally with skin retract

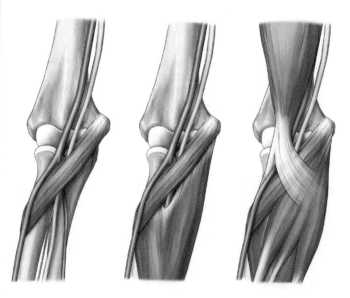

Fig. 11. Relation of the FDS origin, pronator muscle, and median nerve. (*Courtesy of* Julia Ruston, MBBS, London, UK)

but without lengthening the incision, I also cut a part of the lacertus fibrosus. This is conducted not because I feel it has to be cut, but it is easy to do so in the same incision.

Compression to the anterior interosseous nerve (AIN) is another distinct disorder; it is distal to the FDS-pronator syndrome and is rare. With neuritis, the swollen AIN is compressed by surrounding normal structures. Because this nerve is small and no dense structures surround it, a normal AIN is unlikely to be compressed. However, some patients do have tumors or neuropathy, e.g., hourglass-like constriction, compressing the AIN, which should ideally be identified before surgery with ultrasound or MRI scans.[28,29] In these patients, the surgical incision is in the middle of the forearm; the surgeon may or may not include the FDS origin and pronator into exploration or release. AIN neuritis occurs more commonly.[28,30] This is best treated by waiting for many months before contemplating surgery, but if a scan confirms focal compression there is no merit in delaying surgery.

Overall, I do not use a long incision exposing all the median nerves in the middle or proximal forearm and I do not check all sites of possible compression during surgery. The possible sites of compression should largely be excluded through clinical examination and sometimes scans, *before surgery* rather than checking all possible sites during surgery.

In my opinion, these sites can and should be viewed as different disorders. The site of compression can be largely identified preoperatively and surgical exploration is directed to that site. I challenge the need for a large incision; I have been practicing smaller incisions for these problems for many years without disappointment.

CONSIDERATIONS

1. I consider the current nomenclature of the several syndromes of nerve compression should be revised.
2. In my experience, surgical incisions can be small. I challenge the need for large incisions.
3. Inclusion of some sites into regular exploration is a historical misconception. In particular, the ligament of Struthers should not be included routinely in cubital tunnel release.
4. Wide-awake surgery without tourniquet should be used in treating these patients if possible. This approach allows for an intraoperative check of "immediate recovery" of muscle power of the upper extremity, especially in patients with lacertus syndrome or FDS-pronator syndrome.

5. I have no doubt about the existence of these disorders although they are not common.

REFERENCES

1. Granger A, Sardi JP, Iwanaga J, et al. Osborne's ligament: a review of its history, anatomy, and surgical importance. Cureus 2017;9:e1080.
2. Osborne G. Compression neuritis of the ulnar nerve at the elbow. Hand (N Y) 1970;2:10–3.
3. O'Driscoll SW, Horii EM, Carmichael SW, et al. The cubital tunnel and ulnar neuropathy. J Bone Joint Surg Br 1991;73:613–7.
4. Macchi V, Tiengo C, Porzionato A, et al. The cubital tunnel: a radiologic and histotopographic study. J Anat 2014;225:262–9.
5. May-Miller P, Robinson S, Sharma P, et al. The supracondylar process: a rare case of ulnar nerve entrapment and literature review. J Hand Microsurg 2019;11(Suppl 1):S06–10.
6. Tang JB. Ligament of Struthers: exceedingly rarely causes ulnar neuropathy and exploration is not suggested in cubital tunnel syndrome. J Hand Surg Eur 2021;46:800–5.
7. Kane E, Kaplan EB, Spinner M. Sur le trajet du nerf cubital au niveau du bras [Observations of the course of the ulnar nerve in the arm]. Ann Chir 1973;27:487–96.
8. De Jesus R, Dellon AL. Historic origin of the "Arcade of Struthers. J Hand Surg Am 2003;28:528–31.
9. Wehrli L, Oberlin C. The internal brachial ligament versus the arcade of Struthers: an anatomical study. Plast Reconstr Surg 2005;115:471–7.
10. Ochiai N, Hayashi T, Ninomiya S. High ulnar nerve palsy caused by the arcade of Struthers. J Hand Surg Br 1992;17:629–31.
11. Ruiter GCW, de Jonge JGH, Vlak MHM, et al. Ulnar neuropathy caused by muscular arcade of Struthers. World Neurosurg 2020;142:128–30.
12. Sivak WN, Hagerty SE, Huyhn L, et al. Diagnosis of ulnar nerve entrapment at the arcade of Struthers with electromyography and ultrasound. Plast Reconstr Surg Glob Open 2016;4:e648.
13. Lawrence T, Mobbs P, Fortems Y, et al. Radial tunnel syndrome. A retrospective review of 30 decompressions of the radial nerve. J Hand Surg Br 1995;20:454–9.
14. Lister GD, Belsole RB, Kleinert HE. The radial tunnel syndrome. J Hand Surg 1979;4:52–9.
15. McGraw E. Isolated spontaneous posterior interosseous nerve palsy: a review of aetiology and management. J Hand Surg Eur 2019;44:310–6.
16. Moradi A, Ebrahimzadeh MH, Jupiter JB. Radial tunnel syndrome, diagnostic and treatment dilemma. Arch Bone Jt Surg 2015;3:156–62.
17. Portilla Molina AE, Bour C, Oberlin C, et al. The posterior interosseous nerve and the radial tunnel

syndrome: an anatomical study. Int Orthop 1998;22: 102–6.

18. Rekant MS, Wilson MS, Nelson C. Surgery management of compression neuropathies of the elbow. In: Skirven TM, Osterman AL, Fedorczyk JM, et al, editors. Rehabilitation of the hand and upper extremity. 7th Edition. Philadelphia (PA): Elsevier Inc.; 2020.

19. Spinner M. The arcade of Frohse and its relationship to the posterior interosseous nerve entrapment paralysis. J Bone Joint Surg Br 1968;50:809–12.

20. Thomas SJ, Yakin DE, Parry BR, et al. The anatomical relationship between the posterior interosseous nerve and the supinator muscle. J Hand Surg Am 2000;25:936–41.

21. Waljee JF, Fujihara Y, Chung KC. Radial nerve decompression. In: Chung KC, editor. Hand and wrist surgery. 3nd edition. Philadelphia (PA): Elsevier Inc.; 2018. p. 510–4.

22. Xiao TG, Cartwright MS. Ultrasound in the evaluation of radial neuropathies at the elbow. Front Neurol 2019;10:216.

23. Tang JB. Radial tunnel syndrome: definition, distinction and treatments. J Hand Surg Eur 2020;45: 882–9.

24. Englert HM. Partial fascicular median-nerve atrophy of unknown region. Handchirurgie 1976;8:61–2.

25. Hagert E. Clinical diagnosis and wide-awake surgical treatment of proximal median nerve entrapment at the elbow: a prospective study. Hand (N Y) 2013;8:41–6.

26. Hagert E, Lalonde D. Nerve entrapment syndromes. In: Neligan, Chang, editors. Plastic surgery. Volume 6. Hand and upper extremity. 4th edition. Philadelphia (PA): Elsevier Inc.; 2018. p. 525–48.

27. Tang JB. Median nerve compression: lacertus syndrome versus superficialis-pronator syndrome. J Hand Surg Eur 2021;46:1017–22.

28. Tang JB. Compression to the anterior interosseous nerve is very rare: compression by the normal tissues surrounding it may not exist. J Hand Surg Eur 2022;47:541–2.

29. Leblebicioğlu G. Two clinical observations: pronator syndrome in violinists and anterior interosseous nerve syndrome with pure motor loss. J Hand Surg Eur 2022;47:543–5.

30. Elliot D. Proximal median nerve compressions: anterior interosseous nerve compression - a myth. J Hand Surg Eur 2022;47:540–1.

Discussions About Obstetric Brachial Plexus Injuries

Grey Giddins, MBBCh, FRCS (Orth)[a,b,c,*]

KEYWORDS

- Obstetric brachial plexus injuries • Mechanism of injury • Grading • Surgery
- Nonsurgical treatment • Shoulder • Elbow • Hand

KEY POINTS

- Obstetricians have recently made more progress in obstetric brachial plexus injuries (OBPI) through better prevention than have surgeons with their treatment. Surgeons may be able to help inform the efforts of the obstetricians.
- Much is still disputed or unknown in the treatment of OBPI. The use of the Narakas grading is flawed and unreliable; an alternative grading may help categorize patients better both guiding treatment and helping to compare outcomes.
- The role of early nerve surgery is questioned especially for patients with incomplete injuries.
- Beyondnerve surgery the shoulder is the site of greatest surgical attention yet there remains controversy over the causes and thus the treatment of shoulder contracture.
- Elbow contracture is common but often not very symptomatic. The relatively long lever arms of the humerus and forearm make it amenable to splintage.
- In adulthood secondary surgery and fixed scoliosis seem rare so should not be an indication for compromising treatment during growth.

INTRODUCTION

In this article, I address 6 areas for discussion in the management of patients with obstetric brachial plexus injuries (OBPI) (**Box 1**). I consider these are important areas of debate in the management of these patients but I cannot say they are the most important. Where possible I have referred to the published literature but it is incomplete, and I report on some of my recent experience.

SIX AREAS OF DEBATES

What Is the Cause of Obstetric Brachial Plexus Injuries; Does it Matter to the Nerve Surgeon?

The biomechanical cause is a distraction force across the brachial plexus during delivery typically the head/neck distracted away from the shoulder during the second stage of labor. The cause of that force is debated.[1] It had been thought always to be due to the forces applied by the Accoucheur, that is, clinician who delivered the baby. Research in the 1990s showed that OBPI could occur secondary to the forces of the maternal uterus resisted by the maternal birth canal in cases of precipitous births whereby the baby is not handled by an Accoucheur before delivery; I have seen such a case. In all of these reported cases, the nerve injury was incomplete and temporary with full recovery. It was possible that the forces of the maternal uterus could be causing permanent nerve injuries but it was not known as there was always handled by the Accoucheur at a difficult delivery. Professor Draycott and colleagues[1] in Bristol in UK have shown that with optimal care almost all permanent OBPI can be avoided in cases of shoulder dystocia, implying that the

[a] The Hand to Elbow Clinic, Bath, United Kingdom; [b] Royal United Hospital, Bath, United Kingdom;
[c] University of Bath, Bath, United Kingdom
* University of Bath, Bath, United Kingdom.
E-mail address: greygiddins@handtoelbow.com

Hand Clin 38 (2022) 329–335
https://doi.org/10.1016/j.hcl.2022.02.006
0749-0712/22/© 2022 Elsevier Inc. All rights reserved.

Box 1
Some important areas of debates

1. What is the cause of OBPI?

2. Is the Narakas grading of value or reliable?

3. When should surgeons undertake nerve surgery?

4. What is the cause of shoulder tightness in the patients?

5. What is the cause of elbow flexion contracture/radial head dislocation? How can we improve it?

6. Do these patients need surgery in adulthood?

forces of the maternal uterus are rarely if ever strong enough to cause permanent OBPI at shoulder dystocia.

There are, however, cases of OBPI whereby the injury has occurred on the side of the posterior shoulder at delivery. It is considered this is due to the forces of the maternal uterus resisted by the posterior shoulder impacting in the birth canal typically on the maternal sacral promontory. In breach deliveries the mechanism seems to be a distraction force presumably from pull on the shoulder away from the neck/head; these babies are typically smaller and often have different patterns of injury from conventional OBPI.

The specifics of the birth injury may not be of interest to surgeons treating OBPI but there are a number of questions remaining that surgeons may help to answer. Obstetricians widely noted that sometimes they have to apply considerable forces at delivery such as with very big babies when the risks of fetal hypoxia have become very high yet no OBPI occurs, but at other times they apply their "normal" forces and a permanent OBPI occurs. While there may be some mis-remembering it is logical to assume that biological variability applies so some babies may be more at risk of permanent OBPI than others. The reasons can only be speculated such as a prefixed brachial plexus (rare), a longer (or shorter) thoracic outlet than normal, a brachial plexus more vulnerable to stretch (perhaps related to relative hypoxia), etc.

While obstetricians and pediatricians see only a few cases in a working lifetime, surgeons in this field may see hundreds so should try to look out for any possible factors that may theoretically increase the risk of OBPI. In addition, the severity of contractures in OBPI, particularly of the shoulder, which is a major cause of morbidity and need for surgery (q.v.) seem unrelated to the severity of the nerve injury. Some other injuries at

birth may occur increasing the risk of contracture, especially around the shoulder and possibly inform prognosis in the early stages. For example, a very rapid delivery by an Accoucheur may do more damage than a slower one, but present in a similar way in the first few months of life. By considering the mechanics of the birth injury in more detail nerve surgeons may be able to help identify higher risk babies or obstetric techniques.

Is the Narakas Grading Still of Value?

A grading in medicine should be reliable, that is, applied and interpreted consistently, useful, that is, in predicting outcome or treatment and validated. I would argue that the Narakas grading[2] is not reliable, its value in predicting the need and benefit from surgery is unproven and not validated. Nonetheless, the recent consensus from a Canadian working group considered that the Narakas grading should be incorporated in the assessment of babies with OBPI.[3]

I have consulted 12 international, experienced nerve surgeons about when and how they undertake the Narakas grading. They report a very variable application of the Narakas grading: some make the assessment within 1 month; others at 3 months; and some never use the grading as they find it so unreliable. Birch[4] considered the Narakas classification valuable; he recommended that it should be applied after about 2 weeks (postdelivery) but most babies are not seen by experts in OBPI at this time so it has to be performed through the interpretation of parental reporting which is unreliable. In addition, some patients have prolonged conduction block and then recover very well making their initial grading unrepresentative of their outcome.

In a review that I have undertaken of 102 patients of permanent OBPI treated and graded by experienced UK surgeons, there were 73 cases with grade I and II injuries; 10 (14%) had a smaller little finger on the side of the injury than on the opposite side indicating an appreciable injury to C8/the lower trunk of the brachial plexus casting doubt on the initial grading as excluding injury to C8/the lower trunk of the brachial plexus. This is logical; it is unrealistic that a stretching injury of the brachial plexus damaging the upper and middle trunks of the brachial plexus will not also injure the lower trunk of the brachial plexus.

This may be considered heresy by some, but I believe Narakas himself, who did so much to advance the study of OBPI, would have favored at least asking the question as to whether his grading remains valuable. Grade II is the commonest grading by far and can be subdivided into 2a and 2b[5] which seem to be a little more reliable based upon assessment at 2 months of age. In the 102 cases of permanent OBPI that I have reviewed in person, all 73 cases of OBPI (grades I and II) had full hand movement (albeit typically with some reduction in strength) while most cases 14 of 18 with complete OBPI (grades III) and all with grade IV injuries had reduced incomplete digital motion and all had incomplete wrist motion; those with grade IV injuries almost always had very poor hand function.

As the prime purpose of the upper limb is to place the hand in space for use, recovery of hand function is critical to the functional outcome of these injured limbs. Therefore, a more useful grading might be into incomplete OBPI, largely Narakas grades I and II, but which acknowledges the potential for some damage to C8/T1/the lower trunk, and complete injuries with the latter divided into less and more severe complete injuries by the presence of a Horner's syndrome, which is a reliable clinical sign. Given the trend toward less nerve surgery in incomplete injuries (q.v.), primary nerve surgery would be reserved mainly for complete injuries meaning research could be undertaken more reliably to assess the role of nerve surgery in a less heterogeneous cohort, that is, of patients with complete OBPI. Moreover, the families of patients could be given more reliable prognoses, that is, that incomplete injuries would be compatible with reasonable hand and upper limb function in most cases and complete injuries will largely lead to patients being predominantly one-handed.

I have measured the grip strength in 93 patients with permanent OBPI aged $\geq$ 5 years. Grip strength was mostly but not always reduced. It was $\geq$ 90% of the contralateral side in 13 cases; 7 of whom had grade 1 injuries and 6 of whom had grade 2 injuries. Grip strength typically, but not completely, followed the severity of the OBPI with a mean grip strength for grade 1 of 84% (range 65%–125%) of the opposite hand, grade 2 of 73% (range 27%–124%), grade 3 of 45% (range 0%–79%) and grade 4 of 19% (range 0%–57%). Of the patients with complete OBPI grades (3 and 4) only 11(32%) had grip strength greater than 25%. Based on ongoing research, when grip strength is less than 25% of the opposite side, there is increasingly limited hand function, especially in the presence of incomplete ranges of hand motion. Thus, most patients with permanent OBPI function predominantly one-handed.

When Should Surgeons Undertake Nerve Surgery?

The enthusiasm for nerve surgery in OBPI has waxed and waned over the greater than 100 years of study of OBPI. Some authors have strongly advocated for surgery in more severe cases (Narakas grades 3 and 4)[6] while other authors have questioned the role of nerve surgery.[7,8] It has been shown that elbow flexion almost always recovers without nerve surgery.[9] I have reviewed the outcomes of 93 patients with permanent OBPI aged $\geq$ 5 years; only 6 (6%) of patients had elbow flexion < grade 4 on the Medical Research Council scale; all but one had had early reconstructive nerve surgery. While these tended to be patients with more severe injuries, this concurs with the published evidence that spontaneous recovery of adequate elbow flexion strength usually occurs even in cases of severe OBPI treated without nerve surgery, meaning that primary nerve grafting in the neck to restore elbow flexion should be avoided not least as there are potential later reconstructive options such as the Oberlin transfer in less severe cases.

The role of surgery to reconstruct nerve function to the shoulder is more debatable. Oberlin[7] has recently argued that it should never be performed as he considers that shoulder function always recovers and there may be a need for later shoulder arthrodesis, although the evidence for this is limited (q.v.). My experience is that shoulder recovery is not as predictable as the recovery of useful elbow flexion. Moreover, the evidence for long-term shoulder pain following OBPI is limited, especially pain sufficient to require surgery in adulthood. A recent long-term follow-up of patients with OBPI suggests that patients with OBPI do not develop further pain into adulthood.[10] That would be logical as although their shoulder joint may have developed imperfectly the 2 sides of the joint will largely be congruent one to the other and an increased risk of degenerative arthritis seems to be more than compensated by underuse due to weakness and stiffness. In addition, there is a clear role for nerve transfers to improve shoulder function, typically with an accessory to suprascapular nerve transfer which seems to give better results than nerve grafting and can be performed after some delay[11] so that waiting for up to a year for recovery seems to have limited downside for patients and their families.

The role of nerve surgery to improve hand function is more debatable. Various surgeons have reported "good" hand function following reconstruction.[12–15] This is largely based on the Raimondi classification.[16] The latter does not include grip strength which is an important component of hand function (q.v.). Nearly full movement but weak grip is of little functional value. In patients of complete OBPI, in particular, when there is a Horner's syndrome, there may be a role for reconstructing the nerves to improve hand function; that should be assessed in well-designed clinical trials not heterogeneous cases series.

What Is the Cause of Shoulder Tightness in Patients with Obstetric Brachial Plexus Injuries?

It has long been held that shoulder tightness into external rotation (ER) OBPI is due to muscle imbalance[17,18] although some authors have questioned that. It seems to me not to address what is observed. Babies often present with shoulder tightness even at an early assessment such $\leq$3 months of age; any adult can overcome the forces of the baby's muscles even when it is crying, yet some of these babies have fixed contracture by 3 months, often earlier. It is very unlikely this will be due to muscle imbalance especially when the parents report undertaking stretches regularly; although it could be argued there is already secondary contracture from muscle imbalance, but that would seem to be very quick.

The classical shoulder contracture in OBPI is an internal rotation (IR) contracture greater in adduction than abduction. I have reviewed the shoulder function in 93 patients with permanent OBPI $\geq$ 5 years old. 84 (90%) had some loss of shoulder ER $\geq 10^0$ loss of range of motion compared with the opposite side always greater in shoulder adduction than abduction. Biomechanically the subscapularis muscle crosses all of the front of the glenohumeral joint and as the center of the muscle (in the scapula) is distal to the center of the glenohumeral joint, the shoulder joint should, in theory, be tighter in abduction than adduction if primarily due to a subscapularis muscle problem. Rather the biomechanics implies a contracture of the upper part of the soft tissues over the front of the shoulder as often seen at open surgical release. Moreover in stretching a baby or child's contracted shoulder into extremal rotation with the shoulder adducted the medial border of the scapula rises also indicating the contracture is in the superior part of the shoulder not uniformly across it.

Recent work has highlighted the loss of shoulder IR.[19] I have also found this in a review of the affected shoulder in 93 patients $\geq$ 5 years old. 86 (92%) had some reduced shoulder IR in abduction (IR 90) of $\geq 10^0$ compared with the opposite side. The proportionate loss of IR as a percentage of the range in the contra-lateral shoulder was greater than the proportionate loss of abduction, flexion, or ER compared with the opposite

(uninjured) shoulder, that is, these patients had on average a greater loss of IR in abduction than any of the other ranges of motion.

Rather than just a loss of movement in one direction typically there seems to be a global shoulder contracture following a permanent OBPI; this fits with the reports of Eismann and colleagues[20] who reported an abduction contracture of the shoulder in OBPI. Exactly why the contracture(s) develops is unclear but as it seems to be global in the shoulder it is presumably related primarily to capsular mal-development following nerve injury. There is also often some superior subscapularis muscle contracture and possibly other muscle problems. Understanding the pathophysiology is important as the shoulder is the commonest site of surgery for OBPI. If the problem is predominantly contracture but is treated as muscle imbalance this is likely to lead to disappointing results although some authors have reported good outcomes just with tendon transfers.[18]

In the 93 patients, I have assessed, there were 43 $\geq$ 10 years old. Of those 32 had had surgery for shoulder IR contracture (a lack of ER), 10 of whom had had revision surgery and 3 had had further Botox injections. Yet 32 of the 43 (74%) patients had active ER in adduction $\leq 20^0$. This implies that the treatment of patient with IR contractures has not been very successful. That may represent a lack of understanding of the pathophysiology of shoulder contractures in OBPI. While I consider that a release of the shoulder joint contractures is the most important part of any operation to improve shoulder ER, I agree with other authors that there may be a role for muscle/tendon transfers to enhance this.[21] As there is almost always an ER contracture, that is, loss of IR, there is likely to be a role for surgery to release posterior shoulder contractures; this is our experience in a small number of cases of arthroscopic posterior capsular release of the shoulder. The shoulder ER contracture (lack of IR) also means that immobilizing patients in ER following anterior shoulder surgery risks further exacerbating any ER contracture so should be avoided or minimized whereby possible. In addition, stretches for babies in the first years of life, as advocated by many experts,[8] should also include stretches into IR; whether this is beneficial is as yet unproven.

What Is the Cause of Elbow Fixed Flexion Contracture/Radial Head Dislocation and How Can We Improve It?

Elbow contracture is also common in permanent OBPI, typically a loss of full extension and often some loss of full flexion. The loss of elbow extension may increase throughout growth as in the shoulder, suggesting that it is a contracture process rather than due to muscle imbalance, that is, the anterior soft tissues are not sufficiently elastic to stretch normally with the forces of growth, so any loss of joint movement will potentially increase with growth, as in the shoulder. This is in distinction to forearm contractures which seem not to change beyond about 5 years of age; in our review of 93 patients with permanent OBPI, forearm contracture was not correlated to elbow contractures.

How these contractures should be treated is unclear.[8] Splints or serial plaster casts can increase elbow extension but, in my experience, often at the loss of some elbow flexion when used in adolescence. Surgery to release elbow contractures has been recommended[22] but only in small case series. At what age the contracture should be addressed and how, that is, splintage or surgery, is unclear. This is unlikely to be answered by further case series.

The cause of the rarer radial head dislocation is unknown. It is also presumably a contracture problem related to biceps tendon/muscle tightness, as opposed to elbow (ulno-humeral) stiffness which is presumably due to anterior elbow capsule or collateral ligament stiffness. Surgery likely causes more problems than benefits as with other chronic radial head dislocations.[23]

Do Patients with Obstetric Brachial Plexus Injuries Need Surgery in Adulthood?

Starting distally in the upper limb there is no evidence that elbow, forearm, wrist, or hand function deteriorates in these patients in adulthood save as a function of aging later in life, or that surgery will help that could not already have been performed in childhood or adolescence, for example, a tendon transfer to improve active wrist extension. While there are case report, there are no large series reported of improved outcomes from surgery to the elbow, forearm, wrist or hand in adulthood for these patients.

There may be a role for trying to improve shoulder movement in adulthood especially if treatment has not been given earlier in life. Surgeons have reported benefit from the Quad procedure in adults[24] and humeral osteotomies to change the shoulder arc of rotation. We have performed arthroscopic shoulder releases in early adulthood with some benefit and minimal morbidity.

The more interesting question seems to be whether there is a need for shoulder surgery related to degeneration secondary to maldevelopment. Without a large prospective cohort study (which does not exist) that question cannot be answered reliably. There are no large published series of the treatment of shoulder pathology in adults with OBPI, which would be expected if this were an uncommon (rather than a rare) problem. Shoulder arthroplasty has been reported in adolescence and early adulthood by Rudge and colleagues[25]; they reported on 9 cases of arthroplasty for OBPI of whom 3 required revision surgery. I have seen 2 patients treated from this unit, both with disappointing results. Seven cases were reported by Werthel and colleagues[26] and one by Gosens and colleagues.[27] Shoulder arthrodesis has been reported in patients with OBPI but only in 35 patients from 1955 to 2019,[28] and one further reports of a technique of arthroscopic shoulder arthrodesis.[29] Overall 53 cases of arthrodesis or arthroplasty of the shoulder have been reported in OBPI. Even allowing for some unreported cases is a tiny number compared with the overall number of cases with permanent OBPI over the last 80 years. It strongly indicates that there is minimal need for shoulder surgery in adults as a result of their OBPI.

In my experience, most patients report some pain with use or with stretches. Among the 26 adult patients I have reviewed with permanent OBPI ($\geq$16 years; mean age 20, range 16–24 years) all reported some discomfort with activity/stretches, but only 8 of 26 reported a background, that is, continuous, ache. In most cases that was mild. In addition, the pain seems to fluctuate and the reported pain was often amenable to simple measures like activity modification. There is logic to considering that the affected glenohumeral joint might become symptomatically arthritic as it will not have developed normally, but the 2 sides of the joint will typically be congruent one to the other unless dislocated. Moreover, the concomitant weakness and stiffness in the affected upper limb will reduce loading on the joint and so be protective. In addition with a weaker and stiffer injured upper limb, most patients do not undertake heavy bimanual tasks or perform more hazardous past-times such as contact sports further protecting their injured shoulder and probably their uninjured contra-lateral upper limb. This is borne out in a recent report of Ploetze and colleagues[10] who reviewed 25 adults with OBPI at a mean age of 44 (range 18–78) years; 13 had had shoulder surgery in childhood. Despite 5 patients having chronic posterior shoulder dislocation and 13 (of 18) having radiographic evidence of osteoarthritis, the mean score for pain was only 2 and none warranted surgical intervention.

Overall it seems that the upper limbs of patients with OBPI are symptomatically static once they reach adulthood. This is important in reassurance and planning for patients with OBPI and avoiding unnecessary follow-up.

There have also been concerns about the development of scoliosis in patients with OBPI. This has been reported by 2 groups[30,31] although a larger series has refuted that.[32] We have reviewed clinically the spines of 93 patients with permanent OBPI aged 5 to 24 years old; there were 49 females and 44 males with a mean age of 12 years. None had fixed scoliosis. Five of the 26 (19%) adults ($\geq$16 years) had a postural thoracic or thoraco-lumbar curve; none was symptomatic. Only 2 of the 67 children (<16 years) had postural scoliosis. It seems that the risk of fixed scoliosis following OBPI is no greater than in the normal population. Thus, patients do not need routine screening and can largely be reassured the risk of fixed scoliosis is very small.

SUMMARY

Overall it could be argued that obstetricians have recently made more progress in OBPI through better prevention than have surgeons with their treatment. Surgeons may be able to help inform the efforts of the obstetricians. There is much that is still disputed or unknown in the treatment of OBPI. The use of the Narakas grading is flawed and unreliable; an alternative grading may help categorize patients better both guiding treatment and helping to compare outcomes. The role of early nerve surgery is being questioned especially for patients with incomplete injuries. Beyond nerve surgery, the shoulder is the site of greatest surgical attention yet there remains controversy over the causes and thus the treatment of shoulder contracture. Given the clinical findings not least the appreciable internal as well as ER stiffness, peri-articular contracture must be important; the role of muscle imbalance is less clear. There is likely to be an increasing role for arthroscopic shoulder contracture release. Elbow contracture is common but often not very symptomatic. The relatively long lever arms of the humerus and forearm make it amenable to splintage. In theory, long-term night splintage from a young age would be beneficial but this is unproven. In adulthood, secondary surgery and fixed scoliosis seem rare so should not be an indication for compromising treatment during growth.

REFERENCES

1. Draycott T, Kubiak K, Arthur E, et al. Causation of permanent brachial plexus injuries to the anterior arm after shoulder dystocia – literature review. J Patient Saf Risk Management 2018;1:1–5.
2. Narakas AO. Obstetric brachial plexus injuries. In: Lamb DW, editor. The paralysed hand. Edinburgh: Churchill Livingstone; 1987. p. 116–35.
3. Coroneos CJ, Voineskos SH, Christakis MK, et al. Obstetrical brachial plexus injury (OBPI): Canada's national clinical practice guideline. BMJ Open 2017;7(1):e014141.
4. Birch R. Obstetric brachial plexus palsy. J Hand Surg Br 2002;27:3–8.
5. Al-Qattan M, El-Sayed AAF, Al-Zahrani AY, et al. Narakas classification of obstetric brachial plexus palsy revisited. J Hand Surg Eur 2009;34:788–91.
6. Pondaag W, Malessy M. Evidence that nerve surgery improves functional outcome for obstetric brachial plexus injury. J Hand Surg Eur 2021;46:229–36.
7. Oberlin C. Rethinking surgical strategy in the management of obstetrical palsy. J Hand Surg Eur 2021;46:705–7.
8. Hems T. Questions regarding natural history and management of obstetric brachial plexus palsy. J Hand Surg Eur 2021;46:796–9.
9. Hems TEJ, Savaridas T, Sherlock DA. The natural history of recovery of elbow flexion after obstetric brachial plexus injury managed without nerve repair. J Hand Surg Eur 2017;42:706–9.
10. Ploetze K, Goldfarb C, Roberts S, et al. Radiographic and clinical outcomes of the shoulder in long-term follow-up of brachial plexus birth injury. J Hand Surg Am 2020;45:1115–22.
11. Nickel KJ, Morzycki A, Hsiao R, et al. Nerve transfer is superior to nerve grafting for suprascapular nerve reconstruction in obstetrical brachial plexus birth injury: a meta-analysis. 15589447211030691. Hand (N Y) 2021. https://doi.org/10.1177/15589447211030691. Online ahead of print.
12. Birch R, Ahad N, Kon H, et al. Repair of obstetric brachial plexus palsy; results in 100 children. J Bone Joint Surg Br 2005;87:1089–95.
13. Haerle M, Gilbert A. Management of complete obstetric brachial plexus lesions. J Paediatr Orthop 2004;24:194–200.
14. Maillet M, Romana C. Complete obstetric brachial plexus palsy; surgical improvement to recover a functional hand. J Child Orthop 2009;3:101–8.
15. Pondaag W, Malessy M. Recovery oof hand function following nerve grafting and transfer in obstetric brachial plexus lesions. J Neurosurg 2006;105:33–40.
16. Raimondi P. Evaluation of results in obstetric brachial plexus palsy: the hand. Presented at International Meeting on Obstetric Brachial Plexus Palsy, Heerlen, The Netherlands. 1993
17. Bahm J, Wein B, Alhares G, et al. Assessment and treatment of glenohumeral joint deformities in

children suffering from obstetric brachial plexus palsy. J Ped Orthop B 2007;16:243–51.

18. Ozben H, Atalar AC, Bilsel K, et al. Transfer of latissimus dorsi and teres major tendons without subscapularis release for the treatment of obstetrical brachial plexus palsy sequela. J Shoulder Elbow Surg 2011;20:1265–74.

19. Delioglu K, Uzumcugil A, Öztürk E, et al. Relative importance of factors affecting activity and upper extremity function in children with Narakas Group 2 brachial plexus birth palsy. J Hand Surg Eur 2021; 46:239–46.

20. Eismann EA, Little K, Laor T, et al. Glenohumeral abduction contracture in children with unresolved neonatal brachial plexus palsy. J Bone Joint Surg Am 2015;97:112–8.

21. Sibinski M, Hems TEJ, Sherlock DA. Management strategies for shoulder reconstruction in obstetric brachial plexus injury with special reference to loss of internal rotation after surgery. J Hand Surg Eur 2012;37:772–9.

22. Gilbert A. Obstetrical brachial plexus palsy. In: Tubiana R, editor. Hand4. Philadelphia (PA): WB Saunders; 1993. p. 575–601.

23. Huo CW. Radial head dislocation as a rare complication of obstetric brachial plexus palsy: literature review and five case series. Hand Surg 2012;17: 33–6.

24. Nath RK, Goel D, Somasundaram C. Clinical and functional outcome of modified Quad surgery in adult obstetric brachial plexus injury patients: case reports. Clin Pract 2019;9:1140.

25. Rudge WB, Sewell MD, Al-Hadithy N, et al. Shoulder linked arthroplasty in patients with obstetric brachial plexus palsy can improve quality of life and function at short-term follow-up. J Shoulder Elbow Surg 2015; 24:1473e1480.

26. Werthel JD, Schoch B, Frankle M, et al. Shoulder arthroplasty for sequelae of obstetric brachial plexus injury. J Hand Surg Am 2018;43:871.

27. Gosens T, Neumann L, Wallace WA. Shoulder replacement after Erb's palsy: a case report with ten years' follow-up. J Shoulder Elbow Surg 2004; 13:568–72.

28. Belkheyar Z, Belkacem Djeffel A, Cambon-Binder A, et al. Glenohumeral fusion in adults with sequelae of obstetric brachial plexus injury: a report of eight cases. J Hand Surg Eur 2019;44:248–55.

29. Morsy M, Gawish HM, Galal MA, et al. Arthroscopic shoulder fusion for obstetric brachial plexus palsy. Arthrosc Tech 2020;9:e1049–55.

30. Candan AS, Firat T, Livanelioglu A. Assessment of spinal curvatures in children with upper trunk obstetrical brachial plexus palsy. Paediatr Phys Ther 2019; 31:149–54.

31. Partridge C, Edwards S. Obstetric brachial plexus palsy: increasing disability and exacerbation of symptoms with age. Physiother Red Int 2004;9: 157–93.

32. Strömbeck C, Krumlinde-Sundholm L, Remahl S, et al. Long-term follow-up of children with obstetric brachial plexus palsy I: functional aspects. Dev Med Child Neurol 2007;49:198–203.

Direct Repair of Flexor Tendons Close to Bony Insertion and Ruptured Collateral Ligaments

Jin Bo Tang, MD

KEYWORDS

- Bone-tendon junction • Collateral ligaments • Sagittal band of the extensor tendons
- Surgical repair • Direct repair • Grafting

KEY POINTS

- Lacerated flexor tendons close to their inserting can be repaired with robust direct suture repair without pullout sutures.
- Subacute or chronic traumatic ruptures of the midpart of the collateral ligaments can also be repaired by refreshing the lacerated ligament ends and repairing them with multiple sutures together with tightening the elongated joint capsule, thus avoiding the need for a tendon graft.
- Chronic sagittal band injuries with subluxation of the extensor tendons secondary to central slip failure can be repaired with debridement of the central slip tendon and direct repair without a tendon graft to stabilize the central slip.

INTRODUCTION

I chose to discuss the following topics to challenge current surgical beliefs. I have used direct suture repairs of the terminal flexor tendon to very short distal residual tendon stumps attaching them to the distal phalanx instead of a pullout suture. I have also repaired ruptured collateral ligaments of the thumb metacarpophalangeal (MP) joint weeks or months after injury with direct suture repair avoiding tendon grafting. Similarly, I repair the ruptured central slip to local tissues in cases with subluxation of the sagittal band to help reduce the tendon subluxation again avoiding the need for tendon grafting.

I have learnt that some other surgeons also treat these disorders similarly. I present the surgical indications and methods, as well as arguments about the use in more patients than currently considered.

FLEXOR TENDON CUT CLOSE TO TENDON-BONE JUNCTION

Surgical Methods

I consider it possible to directly repair digital flexor tendons (flexor digitorum profundus or flexor pollicis longus) cut close to the tendon-bone junction, that is, in zone 1A (Fig. 1).[1,2] I use a robust end-to-end repair, with 10 or 12 strands of 4-0 nylon sutures to connect the proximal tendon to the very short distal tendon stump, the periosteum of the distal phalanx, and sometimes a part of the distal volar plate of the distal interphalangeal (DIP) joint (Fig. 2).[2]

I start with a 2-strand Kessler repair starting the suture in the proximal stump. I supplement this with several 2-strand repairs with a rectangular configuration (see Fig. 2) of different lengths including other local tissues such as periosteum and the distal volar plate in the distal sutures.

Department of Hand Surgery, Affiliated Hospital of Nantong University, Nantong, Jiangsu, China
E-mail address: jinbotang@yahoo.com

Hand Clin 38 (2022) 337–341
https://doi.org/10.1016/j.hcl.2022.02.004
0749-0712/22/© 2022 Elsevier Inc. All rights reserved.

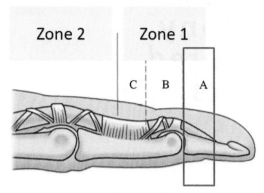

Fig. 1. The injury in flexor tendon zone 1A is the tendon distal to the DIP joint. The distal stump is very short when the tendon is cut in zone 1A- British

The suture methods used for such a direct repair can be variable. However, it is important that the repair should be very strong, which creates tight junction of the proximal tendon end to the residual stump distally. Any other soft tissues located close to the tendon-bone junction can be used for suture purchase. I consider it is critical to have at least 10 strands in the repair (**Fig. 3**).

After completion of surgical repair, I perform digital extension-flexion test similarly as I do for zone 2 repair.[3–6] During this test, I pay more attention to the repair during digital extension and ensure no gapping at all at the repair site. In most patients, I ensured no obvious elongation at the repair site and the repair site was very firm after the robust multistrand repair.

I have not used a pullout suture for almost a decade and consider the strong direct repair works very well. The pullout sutures involve more complex surgical procedures, can cause potential damage to nails, needs secondary suture removal, and risks infection down the suture track.

Postoperative Care

After surgery, I immobilize the digits with a dorsal plaster splint in mild flexion for 2 weeks without undertaking any finger/thumb movement (**Fig. 4**); I start passive motion of the digits from the beginning of week 3. From the beginning of week 5, patients are instructed to do active flexion exercises. In week 6, the splint can be discarded or only used part-time such as when going out or in the night.

Passive motion after 2 weeks is primarily to prevent or reduce finger stiffness. The number of sessions and duration of each session for passive motion in weeks 3 and 4 are similar to motion exercises used after flexor tendon repairs in zone 2.[7] I ensure that the patient exercises 4 to 6 sessions a day. Each exercise session lasts 15 to 20 minutes,

which ensures at least 40 runs of motion in each session.[7] The patient performs exercise at home according to my instruction at first, third, and sixth week after surgery in clinic follow-up.

Because the repair site is distal to the DIP joint, I do not worry about adhesion formation as they should not affect digital flexion but should enhance healing of the repair site. I consider this is enhanced by avoiding any motion in the first 2 weeks after surgery. The healing of the repaired sites is usually strong enough for active motion from week 5, and return to normal hand use should be from weeks 9 or 10 after surgery.

COLLATERAL LIGAMENTS OF THE THUMB MP JOINTS

A tendon graft is often recommended for chronic disruption of the collateral ligament of the thumb MP joint. I perform a direct reinforced repair of the collateral ligament. I have not used a tendon graft unless there is a substantial defect in the ligament (**Fig. 5**). Other surgeons also have reported direct repair for the chronic cases of collateral ligament disruption.[8,9]

Many surgeons perhaps consider tendon graft is indicated in these patients.[10–12] I suspect that the recommendation for tendon grafting is based on the belief that a ruptured ligament does not have sufficient healing potential when the site of injury is no longer fresh. As the healing potential of a lacerated tendon or ligament is widely recognized,[13–15] the need of a graft to repair chronic disruption of collateral ligaments may need revising.

Without a defect, direct repair of the ruptured ligament can be expected to heal when the ruptured ends of the ligament are "freshened up" during surgery. A key step is to debride the area of the collateral ligament division sufficiently to refresh both stumps of the ligament in order to promote optimal healing. Because the joint capsule is often loose in these patients, I add reinforcing sutures to repair/tighten the joint capsule in the area of the ligament rupture (see **Fig. 5**).

After surgery, the thumb MP joint is protected with a splint in full extension for 3 weeks to allow early healing; after that, the splint is removed for passive and active partial (up to 50%) range of joint flexion to reduce joint stiffness.[7] The partial range of motion helps protect the repair.[7] The repaired ligament gradually regains elasticity after passive and active motion. A splint should be used to protect the repair for a minimum of 4 or 5 weeks from surgery. Full range of flexion is allowed about 5 to 6 weeks after surgery, after which full range of flexion gradually recovers.

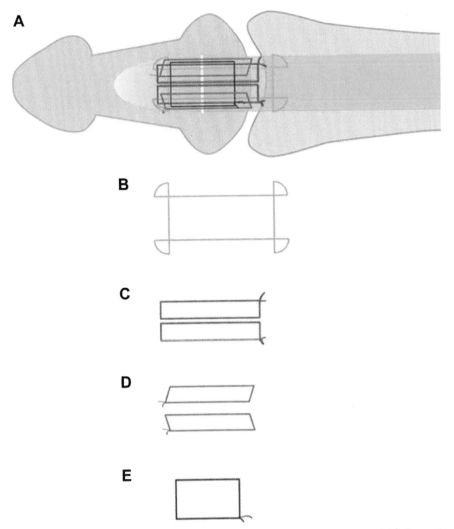

Fig. 2. A drawing showing a robust direct repair with a 12-strand core suture that I used for the patients. (*Adapted from* Wu YF, Tang JB. Letter regarding "A 10- or 12 strand core suture in a flexor tendon in zones I, II, and III". J Hand Surg Am. 2015;40(12):2510-2511. https://doi.org/10.1016/j.jhsa.2015.08.031; with permission.)

I have repaired the traumatic disruption of the collateral ligaments directly on average 2 or 3 times each year over the last decade. I have been pleased with the results with no cases requiring secondary tendon grafting. I consider the graft reconstruction is much more difficult to perform and may not give as good an outcome.

In patients with a substantial defect of a disrupted collateral ligament where direct approximation of the disrupted ligament likely is difficult and a graft may be necessary but this is infrequent in my experience.

SAGITTAL BAND/CENTRAL SLIP INJURIES

Similarly, I repair the chronic sagittal band/central slip injuries with subluxation of the extensor tendons over the MP joint with debridement of the site of injury and direct suture repair of the sagittal band/central slip after reduction of the subluxation of the extensor tendon; I do not use a tendinous band or tendon graft to reinforce/reconstruct the extensor tendon over the MP joint (distal to the MP joint the extensor tendon continues as the central slip). The direct repair without a tendinous band to stabilize the central slip has been used for a patient without bony deformity of the MP joint. I use 4-0 monofilament nylon suture or 4-0 braided suture (such as Ethibond) to make figure-of-eight repair or simple direct repair.

After surgery, I splint the finger in full or almost full extension for 3 to 4 weeks followed by partial range of active flexion exercise for a few weeks.

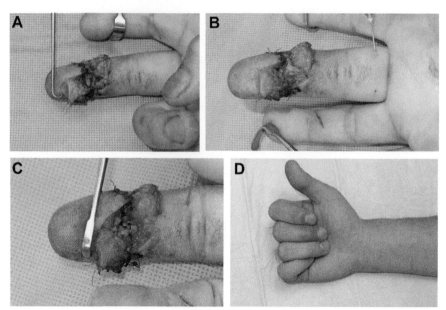

Fig. 3. (*A*) A patient with traumatic cut at the terminal area of the flexor digitorum profundus (FDP) tendon in zone 1A. (*B*) The retracted proximal FDP tendon stump was brought into the site of the cut through an incision in the palm and pushing the retracted FDP tendon distally with 2 sets of forceps. (*C*) Surgical repair with a 10-strand repair, with attachment of distal anchor to tendon stump and periosteum etc. (*D*) Functional outcomes at week 8 after surgery (copyright, Jin Bo Tang, MD, Jiangsu, China).

The range of active flexion-extension gradually increases in subsequent weeks. The number of sessions and duration of each session are similar to those after flexor tendon repair[7]; the patient's exercise is less stringent if the repair site is not large or surgical repair is strong. The timing of starting the exercise after extensor tendon repair can be at 3 or 4 weeks after surgery, which is much later than after flexor tendon repair. Depending on the severity of extensor tendon disruption, the exercise regime needs adjustment.

CONSIDERATIONS AND SUMMARY
Considerations for Surgical Indications and Technical Keys

1. I recommend direct multistrand suture repair of the flexor tendon in zone 1A close to tendon-

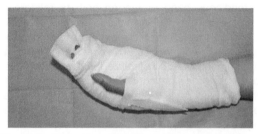

Fig. 4. Postoperative protection of the repaired finger in mild flexion with a dorsal plaster splint for 2 weeks without motion, followed by passive motion for 2 weeks, and then active finger flexion exercise.

bone junction; I do not use a pullout suture. Any tissues around the insertion site of the distal tendon can be used for anchoring the sutures as well as the short distal tendon stump.
2. For direct repair of the ruptured thumb MP joint collateral ligament, I stress the need for freshening up the injury site and tightening the joint capsule near the site of the collateral ligament disruption.
3. I consider it is better to repair the ligament too tight than too loose as the repair site will typically allow recovery of motion range postoperatively during rehabilitation.

Considerations About Postoperative Protection and Motion

1. Following distal suture repair of zone 1 flexor tendon, I immobilize the digit for the first 2 weeks, allow passive motion from weeks 3 to 4, then start active flexion exercise from week 5.
2. Following collateral ligament repair, I immobilize for 3 weeks but thereafter quickly introduce passive and active partial rang joint motion.

Future Attention and Exploration

I urge other surgeons to consider simpler direct repair and to define the situations in which a direct repair can safely replace complex procedures. There have been reports in recent years about the

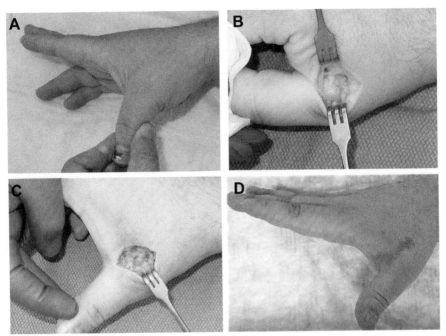

Fig. 5. (*A*) A patient with chronic gamekeeper's thumb. (*B*) Surgery revealed disruption of the ulnar collateral ligament with scar formation. (*C*) 3-0 Ethibond was used to make a very tight repair when the thumb MP joint was held in full extension. (*D*) Postoperative recovery of stable MP joint without laxity and radial deviation during thumb motion (copyright, Jin Bo Tang, MD, Jiangsu, China).

treatment of collateral ligament injuries; I consider they overemphasize the need of tendon grafting procedures. I recommend direct repair as an alternative. Future studies should attend to effective, less complicated methods for these injuries and in particular to define the indications for direct suturing or tendon grafting in treating collateral ligament injury of the thumb MP joint and the MP joint of fingers.

REFERENCES

1. Moiemen NS, Elliot D. Primary flexor tendon repair in zone 1. J Hand Surg Br 2000;25:78–84.

2. Wu YF, Tang JB. Letter regarding "A 10- or 12-strand core suture in a flexor tendon in zones I, II, and III. J Hand Surg Am 2015;40:2510–1.

3. Tang JB. Outcomes and evaluation of flexor tendon repair. Hand Clin 2013;29:251–9.

4. Tang JB, Zhou X, Pan ZJ, et al. Strong digital flexor tendon repair, extension-flexion test, and early active flexion: experience in 300 tendons. Hand Clin 2017;33:455–63.

5. Tang JB. Recent evolutions in flexor tendon repairs and rehabilitation. J Hand Surg Eur 2018;43:469–73.

6. Tang JB, Lalonde D, Harhaus L, et al. Flexor tendon repair: recent changes and current methods. J Hand Surg Eur 2022;47:31–9.

7. Tang JB. Rehabilitation after flexor tendon repair and others: a safe and efficient protocol. J Hand Surg Eur 2021;46:813–7.

8. Christensen T, Sarfani S, Shin AY, et al. Long-term outcomes of primary repair of chronic thumb ulnar collateral ligament injuries. Hand (N Y). 2016;11:303–9.

9. Agout C, Bacle G, Brunet J, et al. Chronic instability of the thumb metacarpo-phalangeal joint: Seven-year outcomes of three surgical techniques. Orthop Traumatol Surg Res 2017;103:923–6.

10. Fairhurst M, Hansen L. Treatment of "Gamekeeper's Thumb" by reconstruction of the ulnar collateral ligament. J Hand Surg Br 2002;27:542–5.

11. Schroeder NS, Goldfarb CA. Thumb ulnar collateral and radial collateral ligament injuries. Clin Sports Med 2015;34:117–26.

12. Ritting AW, Baldwin PC, Rodner CM. Ulnar collateral ligament injury of the thumb metacarpophalangeal joint. Clin J Sport Med 2010;20:106–12.

13. Manske PR. Flexor tendon healing. J Hand Surg Br 1988;13:237–45.

14. Boyer MI. Flexor tendon biology. Hand Clin 2005;21:159–66.

15. Wu YF, Tang JB. Tendon healing, edema, and resistance to flexor tendon gliding: clinical implications. Hand Clin 2013;29:167–78.

Fig. 5. (A) A patient with chronic rupture of the flexor pollicis longus. (B) Surgery revealed disruption of the distal lateral ligament with sutures. (C) Bioabsorbable screws used to reconnect the thumb. (D) Postoperative recovery of thumb motion comparison. (Jin Bo Tang, MD, Jiangsu, China)

REFERENCES

Our Disagreement on "Iceberg View" on the Ulnar Wrist and Clinical Implications

Eduardo R. Zancolli III, MD

KEYWORDS

- Ulnar • Wrist • Distal radioulnar joint • Triquetrolunate joint • Triquetrohamate joint
- Pisotriquetral joint • Ligament • Surgery

INTRODUCTION

During the last decades, we have witnessed a huge interest in pathologies of the ulnar side of the wrist. Many advances (biomechanical, diagnostic, arthroscopic, and surgical) have been achieved particularly in the assessment and treatment of the distal radioulnar joint (DRUJ) and the lunotriquetral joint (LTJ). Even so, when we critically analyze the results we find that a significant percentage of patients do not have pain-free wrists and a full return to previous activities, and we highlight that pain is usually the main or only presenting symptom.

Considering the triangular ligament, we can find papers such as the multicenter study that revealed residual postoperative pain in 36% of the patients.[1] When we analyze LT instability we find no better surgical outcomes. Marc García-Elías, (personal communication) analyzed 9 papers on the treatment of LT instability; he concluded that an average of 39% of the operated cases did not achieve a pain-free wrist.

Residual pain is the main problem to address. The main cause of the reported poor outcomes is the incorrect diagnoses often with an incorrect monodiagnosis. This article is to explain our disagreement with an ''iceberg view'' on the ulnar side of the wrist. To consider a new paradigm we must leave aside this usual "iceberg view," that is, considering only what we are seeing above the surface and ignoring what we do not see because it is below it.

The ulnar side of the wrist also includes other areas besides the DRUJ and the LTJ. In particular we are referring to the triquetral-hamate (THJ) and the pisotriquetral joints (PTJ), which are only infrequently reported on in published literature. I suggesst that we reconsider 3 components: (1) the territory of the ulnar side; (2) the biomechanics; and (3) the grades of instability.

THE UNDERWATER PART OF THE ICEBERG: 3 COMPONENTS
The Territory of the Ulnar Side

As well as the DRUJ and LTJ we need to consider the PTJ and THJ. The PTJ has been reported on rarely; there are reports of complete dislocations of the triquetrum[2] and the pisiform[3,4] but we could find only one paper[5] referring to pathology at the PTJ in racquet players. Current knowledge attributes most cases of midcarpal instability to the LTJ. But when considering the ulnar side territory it would seem strange to have pathology only in 2 areas (DRUJ and LTJ) and not in the other 2 (THJ and PTJ).

New Biomechanical Considerations

Our understanding of wrist pathology based in part on models; the main biomechanical model that we have for understanding the ulnar side is the Columnar Theory of Navarro/Taleisnik.[6,7] It is helpful but may be too basic for the interpretation of the different possible lesions. For carpal instability we

Argentine Association for Hand Surgery Specialists' Career, Barriexos 1584 – 13A, Buenos Aires 1115, Argentina
E-mail address: eduardozancolli@gmail.com

Hand Clin 38 (2022) 343–350
https://doi.org/10.1016/j.hcl.2022.04.001
0749-0712/22/© 2022 Elsevier Inc. All rights reserved.

also have the models of Mayfield and colleagues.[8] I consider that a similar concept could be applied to the ulnar column.

Based on this analysis, in 2001 we presented a more expanded biomechanical model: the "peritriquetral lesional ring,"[9] which considers the progression of forces over the ulnar side of the wrist.

As the triquetrum has the greatest number of ligament attachments of the carpal bones, it seems logical that with increasing energy other ulnar structures/areas, around the triquetrum, would be affected, that is, the triangular ligament, the Bourgery ligament[10] (producing extensor carpi ulnaris [ECU] subluxation), the LT ligament, the PT ligament, and the medial TH ligament (**Fig. 1**).

The "dart-throwing" motion,[11,12] the motion from extension-radial deviation to flexion-ulnar deviation, has been shown to be important in daily wrist function. I believe that it should be also studied in the opposite direction, which can be referred to as "inverse dart throwing" (or perhaps more appropriately the "swing arc" of the dart-thrower motion); this is important, as it recognizes the way the midcarpal joint is used in most sports. In tennis, golf, and polo, there is a marked acceleration of the wrist in the inverse dart-throwing direction (swing arc). This swing arc begins in flexion-ulnar deviation and accelerates to extension-radial deviation. This strenuous acceleration must, inevitably, have an end point. I consider it is mainly restrained by the medial side of the THJ. Thus, the medial TH ligament, usually not considered in much detail in current medical literature, has an action as the final limiting structure of this motion.

Grades of Instability: Triquetral-hamate and the Pisotriquetral Joints

Although we report ulnar-sided wrist instability, patients usually report pain, weakness, and reduced function, notably including midcarpal instability.[13–15] We recognize degrees of instability in many joints, often graded as mild, moderate, and severe (or subluxation and dislocation), yet at the PTJ and the THJ we have only seen published reports on dislocations at these joints[2–4]; this begs the question as to why these joints do not also suffer symptomatic instability.

TRIQUETRAL-HAMATE INSTABILITY

From the second half of the 1990s decade, we began identifying pain at the THJ in the dominant wrist of young patients (mean age 28 years). Most of them were tennis, golf, or polo players or professional musicians (71% of our 60 cases). We found that pain at the THJ was usually associated to other ulnar side pathologies (76%), with a median of 2 (range 1–4) associations per wrist. There were 4 common associations and occasionally more than one other pathology: PT instability 62%; triangular fibrocartilage complex (TFCC) lesions 31%; ECU subluxation 19%; and LT instability 12%. We have assessed these problems further.

Anatomy

The THJ has been described as having a complex helicoidal movement, engaging in ulnar deviation and opening in radial deviation. Previous descriptions of the ligaments of the joint refer to the volar TH ligament (the ulnar part of Poirier's "V") but no ligament at the medial side of the joint. In 2001[9] we published our study on the medial hamate ligament and its biomechanical importance, being the limiting structure of the swing arc of the dart thrower's motion movement. It has insertions on the medial side of the triquetrum and the hamate and is reinforced by intimate contact with the floor of the sixth dorsal compartment, thus forming a "ligament-retinaculum complex," limiting excessive opening of the THJ in forced radial deviation. Subsequently we found an earlier report of this ligament by Mizuseki and Ikuta[16] but with no mention of its biomechanical importance or of any associated pathology. Classic anatomic descriptions also do not mention the synovial plica on the medial side of the joint, which can become inflamed. E. A. Zancolli with C. Zaidenberg, also studied this complex reporting that the floor of the sixth dorsal compartment has a 9 mm insertion into the triquetrum and 5 mm insertion into the hamate (**Fig. 2**).

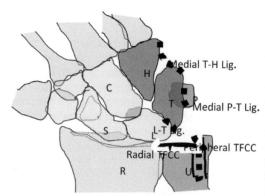

Fig. 1. "Peritriquetral lesional ring" and the ulnar side possible associations according to the lesional energy: TFCC radial to peripheral; Bourgery ligament (ECU subluxation); LT ligament; PT ligament, and medial TH ligament.

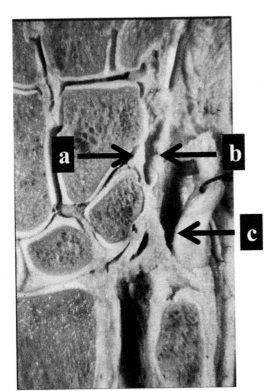

Fig. 2. Anatomy. a. Medial TH ligament; b. reinforcement by the floor of the sixth dorsal compartment; c. ECU retracted with a hook. (*Courtesy of* E. A. Zancolli II, MD, Buenos Aires, Argentina.)

Clinical Features

In our experience patients with THJ instability present with diffuse pain in their dominant wrist while performing their demanding sportive or musical activities, typically not well localized to a specific site on the ulnar side of their wrist. They usually report that the pain disappears shortly after finishing their activity. None reported instability. Except for 2 severe and chronic cases, none reported rest pain or pain from non–weight-bearing activities.

It is interesting to note that when pain was present it was not related to the THJ but to other ulnar associated pathologies, for example, DRUJ pain.

Physical Examination

Meticulous palpation should reveal tenderness over the medial side of the THJ; this is exacerbated by moving the wrist from radial to ulnar deviation. We consider this pain is due to an impingement of the plica when the THJ "engages." We confirm the relevance of the tenderness by asking patients whether it provokes the pain they suffer. If in doubt we ask patients to perform their provocative activity immediately before the next consultation.

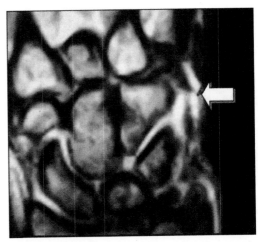

Fig. 3. MRI: disruption of the medial TH complex (*arrow*).

Complementary Studies

We have found that standard radiographs and CT scans are not useful for diagnosis. MRI and midcarpal arthrography, done separately to avoid missing inflammatory fluid on the medial side of the hamate, are the most useful investigations. The T2 fat suppression coronal MRI scan views show disruption of the normal anatomy of the medial complex THJ (**Fig. 3**) and an inflamed/hypertrophic plica (**Fig. 4**). Axial views show the presence of fluid in the medial part of the hamate at the

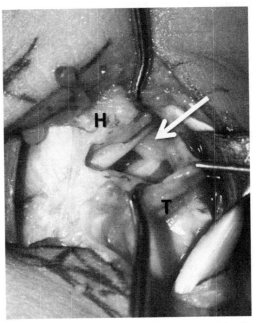

Fig. 4. Intraoperative: inflamed TH synovial plica (*arrow*).

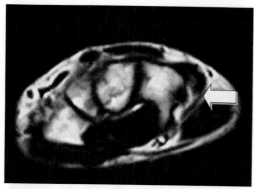

Fig. 5. MRI: contrast solution on the medial side of the hamate-rupture of distal insertion (*arrow*).

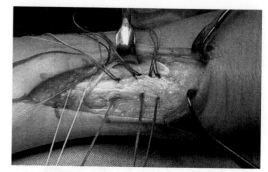

Fig. 7. Augmentation with the ECU tendon.

site of the distal insertion of the ligament complex (**Fig. 5**). Midcarpal arthrography reveals an increase of the contrast solution at the TH recess and, sometimes, passage of the contrast into the little finger carpomtecarpal joint.

Treatment

All patients are initially treated with conservative treatment: ice, nonsteroidal antiinflammatory drugs (NSAIDs), splinting, and physiotherapy. If at 3 to 4 weeks they have not improved, a steroid injection is given into the THJ. If symptoms persist thereafter surgery is recommended.

Surgical technique

Because of a lack of described surgical techniques for this joint, we have designed a technique for reconstructing the medial hamate ligament complex with plication and augmentation.[9]

When this is the only ulnar pathology to be treated or treatment is combined with treating PT instability, we use a skin incision following the direction of the dorsal cutaneous branch of the ulnar

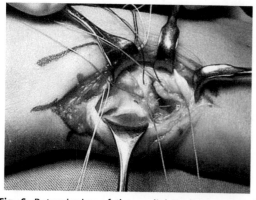

Fig. 6. Retensioning of the medial TH ligament and sixth dorsal compartment floor in one plane.

nerve, ending at the dorsoulnar angle at the base of the little finger metacarpal (MC). When surgery for TH instability is combined with surgery to the TFCC, we start the incision dorsally over the center of the ulnar head ending at the same point as the aforementioned incision. The dorsal cutaneous branch of the ulnar nerve is identified and protected. Next, the roof of the sixth dorsal compartment is opened longitudinally over approximately 3 cm and the ECU tendon retracted ulno-volarly. For security, a small longitudinal incision is made over the fifth dorsal compartment to identify and protect the extensor digiti minimi tendon. Using a small needle (23 or 25 gauge) the articular space of the THJ is identified. The THJ is opened through floor of the sixth dorsal compartment via the medial TH ligament (**Fig. 6**) and capsule using an oblique incision following the direction of the joint (dorsal-proximal to volar-distal with an approximate inclination of 25°–30°).

After removing the plica, the medial structures are plicated in neutral ulnar deviation using absorbable 3/0 sutures. If the tissues are plicated in ulnar deviation, radial deviation will be lost postoperatively. The repair of the medial structures is augmented with the ECU tendon (**Fig. 7**). An incision is made to the deep surface of the ECU tendon (up to 50% of the tendon width) to create a flat tendon face overlying the plication. The ECU is sutured on top of the plication using the same absorbable sutures. The goal is to have an active ECU tendon up to the triquetrum but functioning as a tenodesis to the base of the little finger MC.

Postoperative care

The wrist is immobilized in a short arm plaster cast for 4 weeks, then supported in a removable wrist splint for another 4 weeks with intermittent active and passive exercises. At 6 weeks postoperatively radial and ulnar deviation exercises are begun. At 8 weeks strengthening exercises are started and at 4 months potsoperatively patients are allowed

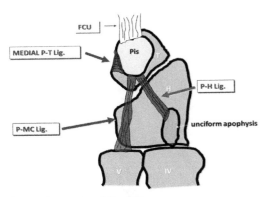

Fig. 8. Ligaments of the PTJ.

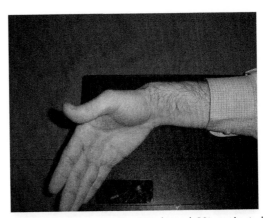

Fig. 10. Incidence for the PTJ: lateral 20° supinated with 20° wrist flexion.

to return to sport. In cases where the TFCC is also repaired an aforementioned elbow plaster cast is applied for the first 4 weeks.

PISOTRIQUETRAL INSTABILITY

Even though the anatomy of some of the ligaments of the PTJ has been described,[17–19] the bibliography reporting pisotriquetral instability is scarce for even when the pisiform bone is removed.[20–22] I would ask why remove the pisiform and not perform a ligament reconstruction as for other joint instability? In 1996 E. A. Zancolli presented a paper on PTJ instability at the Kleinert Institute[23,24] and in 2004 I presented a paper on this topic at the IFSSH Congress.[25]

Anatomy

The pisiform is stabilized, longitudinally by 2 ligaments, the pisohamate ligament (PHL), from the pisiform to the unciform apophysis and the pisometacarpal ligament (PML), from the pisiform to the base of the little finger MC (volarly) (**Fig. 8**).

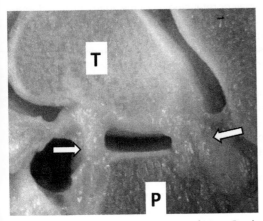

Fig. 9. Medial PT ligament. (*Courtesy of* Marc Garcia-Elias, MD PhD, Barcelona, Spain.)

They prevent proximal dislocation of the pisiform with contraction of the flexi carpi ulnaris (FCU).

Zancolli described a third ligament, the medial pisotriquetral ligament.[23,24] This ligament prevents excessive opening in an anteroposterior plane between the pisiform and the triquetrum. I presented a paper on this instability at the ninth Congress of the IFSSH[25] in 2004, and in 2005 Rayan and colleagues[26,27] presented papers studying the ligaments but called the medial ligament the "ulnar" PT ligament (**Fig. 9**).

Symptoms

Patients can present with isolated PTJ problems or problems associated with other ulnar-sided pathology, for example, the DRUJ. They usually present with pain with demanding activities but sometimes also with daily life activities that demand active contraction of the FCU. The symptoms are typically in their dominant hand.

Physical Examination

Meticulous physical examination reveals localized pain at the ulnar side of the PTJ when palpating with the examiner's thumb. When pain is elicited with this maneuver the patient should be asked if that reproduces the pain they are reporting.

Imaging Studies

The key tests are radiographs and an MRI scan. Radiographs are performed with a lateral view, 20° supinated (**Fig. 10**) or tangential to Lister tubercle.[28] This view allows measurement of opening of the PTJ. Jameson and colleagues[29] established that the mean opening of the normal, unloaded PTJ is 0.5 mm. They also studied that same view but with 20° of wrist flexion (**Fig. 11**) reporting a mean opening of 3.5 mm. We have

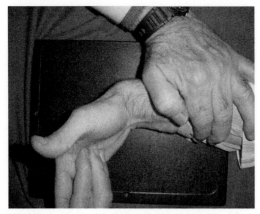

Fig. 11. Same incidence but with resisted wrist flexion.

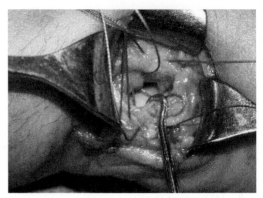

Fig. 13. The medial PT ligament after local synovectomy.

added an extra study, resisting wrist flexion (**Fig. 12**). In our experience a gap of more than 3.5 mm is pathologic. Patients with increased ligamentous laxity may have an opening of more than 3.5 mm; we perform comparative radiographs of the opposite side.

The T2 axial MRI scan views with fat suppression show elongation or disruption of the medial PT ligament and increased fluid in the joint.

Pathology and Classification

In minor or moderate instabilities the only affected structure is the medial PT ligament. In a severe instability not only is that ligament compromised but also the PHL and the PML. When both are defunctioned proximal dislocation of the pisiform is shown on unloaded radiographs.

Based on these factors we have proposed the following classification:

Type I: pathologic medial opening (medial PT ligament injury)

Type II: pathologic medial opening with proximal translation of the pisiform (subluxation or dislocation) (medial PT + PH + PM ligament injuries)

Treatment

As with TH instability all patients are initially treated with conservative treatment: ice, NSAIDs, splinting, and physiotherapy. If at 3 to 4 weeks they have not improved, a steroid injection is given into the THJ. If symptoms persist thereafter surgery is recommended.

Surgical technique

I consider that all the affected ligaments should be repaired. For type 1 instabilty on its own the skin incision is made following the dorsal cutaneous branch of the ulnar nerve. If associated with DRUJ instability, the incision begins dorsally, that is, radial to the ECU and is directed in a smooth "S" shape distal to the medial side of the little finger MC. The dorsal cutaneous branch is found and protected. The dorsal retinaculum is cut transversally volar to the PTJ and carefully elevated from volar to dorsal. The PT joint is identified, using a needle or palpation and a transverse incision is made over the medial PT ligament. Once the joint is opened, a synovectomy is usually required. A repair or retensioning of the ligament is performed with 3/0 absorbable sutures (usually 3) at maximum tension; this is augmented with the dorsal retinaculum sutured to the medial ligament using the aforementioned stitches (**Fig. 13**).

In type 2 injuries the medial ligament and the PH ligament are reconstructed. For the latter reconstruction a volar incision is added. The ligament is reconstructed with one-third of the FCU cut proximally and taken and sutured to the unciform apophysis (**Fig. 14**).

Postoperative care

Postoperatively the wrist is immobilized for 4 weeks in a short arm plaster cast, then supported in a removable wrist splint, for another 4 weeks with intermittent active and passive

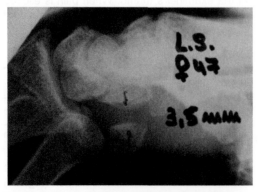

Fig. 12. Incidence showing opening of the PTJ.

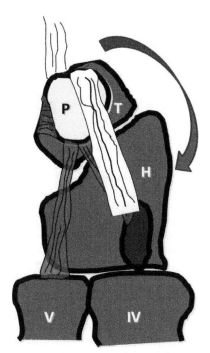

Fig. 14. Reconstruction of the PH ligament with one-third of the FCU.

exercises. At 8 weeks strengthening exercises are started and at 3 months potsoperatively patients are allowed to return to sport. In cases where the TFCC is also repaired an aforementioned elbow plaster cast is applied for the first 4 weeks.

RESULTS AND DISCUSSION

We have explained our view that the problem we are facing with the current paradigm on the ulnar side of the wrist is limiting ourselves to a single diagnosis, in particular believing that only severe instabilities can occur in the TH and PT joints.

We have diagnosed TH instability in 60 wrists and PT instability in 35 wrists. Forty-two percent of patients with THJ and 40% of the patients with PTJ required surgery. We assessed the results of 21 wrist treated for THJ instability with a mean age of 28 years and a mean follow-up of 3 years and 2 months (range 1–7 years) and 14 wrists treated for PTJ instability with mean age of 28 years and with a mean follow-up of 2 years and 8 months (range 1–6 years).[24] Of note, 95% of the THJ and all the PTJ operations were on dominant wrists, and most of the patients practiced demanding sports or were musicians (THJ: 71%; PTJ: 79%). The mean time from onset of symptoms to surgery was 23 months for the THJ and 10 months for the PTJ.

We treat all ulnar-sided pathologies at the same surgical procedure (76% with other ulnar-sided pathologies associated with THJ pathology and 79% associated with PTJ pathology). The triangular ligament was torn or lax in 31% of the patients with THJ instability and in 36% of the patients with PT instability. Of the patients treated for THJ pathology 67% were pain free and 28% had some discomfort; 90% of them returned to their previous activity. Eighty-six percent of patients treated for PTJ instability were pain free with the remainder having some pain but only with mild limitations.

In summary, I believe that we should consider more possible pathologies when assessing ulnar sided wrist pain based on considering (1) the territory of the ulnar side; (2) the biomechanics; and (3) the concept of grades of instability at the THJ and the PTJ.

DISCLOSURE

No conflicts of interest.

REFERENCES

1. Corso SJ, Savoie FH, Geissler WB, et al. Arthroscopic repair of peripheral avulsions of the triangular fibrocartilage complex of the wrist: a multicenter study. Arthroscopy 1997;13:78–84.
2. Braig D, Koulaxouzidis G, Kalash S, et al. Volar dislocation of the triquetrum – case report and review of literature. J Hand Micosurg 2013.
3. Cohen I. Dislocation of the pisiform. Ann Surg 1922; 75:238–9.
4. Immerman EW. Dislocation of the pisiform. J Bone Joint Surg Am 1948;30:489–92.
5. Helal B. Chronic overuse injuries of the pisotriquetral joint in raquet game players. Br J Sports Med 1979;12:195–8.
6. Navarro A. Luxaciones del Carpo. Anales de Fac de Med Montevideo. Orthop Trans 1921;113–41.
7. Taleisnik J. The Ligaments of the Wrist. J Hand Surg Am 1976;1:110–8.
8. Mayfield JK. Pathogenesis of wrist ligament instability. In: Lichtman DM: the wrist and it's disorders. Philadelphia: WB Saunders; 1988. p. 53–73.
9. Zancolli ER III. Localized medial triquetral-hamate instability. Anatomy and operative reconstruction-augmentation. Hand Clinics. Adv Hand Anat 2001; 17:83–96.
10. Bourgery JM, Jacob NA. Traité complet d'anatomie de l'homme. Anatomie descriptive ou phisiologique. H, CA Delanney, Paris. Osteologie et syndesmologie, 2. Miologie; 1832. aponeurologie; 1852.
11. Kane PM, Vopat BG, Mansuripur PK, et al. Relative contributions of midcarpal and radiocarpal joints to

dart-thrower's motion at the wrist. J Hand Surg Am 2018;43:234–40.

12. Kamal RN, Rainbow M, Akelman E, et al. In vivo triquetrum-hamate kinematics through a simulated hammering task wrist motion. J Bone Joint Surg Am 2012;94:e85.

13. Mouchet A, Belot J. Poignet a'ressaut: subluxation mediocarpienne en avant. Bull Memories de la Société Nationale de Chirurgie 1934;60:1243–4.

14. Lichtman DM, Schneider JR, Swafford AR, et al. Ulnar midcarpal instability–clinical and laboratory analysis. J Hand Surg Am 1981;6:515–23.

15. García-Elías M. The non-dissociative clunking wrist: a personal view. J Hand Surg Eur 2008;33:698–711.

16. Mizuseki T, Ikuta Y. The dorsal carpal ligaments: their anatomy and function. J Hand Surg Br 1989;14:91–8.

17. Zancolli EA. Anatomía quirúrgica de la Mano. Atlas ilustrado. Buenos Aires, Argentina: Editorial Médica Panamericana; 2015.

18. Yamaguchi S, Nagao T, Beppu M, et al. Pisotriquetral joint—anatomy and movement. J Jpn Soc Surg Hand 1992;9:25–8.

19. Pevny T, Rayan GM, Egle D. Ligamentous and tendinous support of the pisiform, anatomical and biomechanical study. J Hand Surg Am 1995;20:299–304.

20. Minami M, Yamazaki J, Ishii S. Isolated dislocation of the pisiform: a case report and review of the literature. J Hand Surg Am 1984;9:125–7.

21. Carroll RE, Coyle MP. Dysfunction of the pisotriquetral joint: treatment by excision of the pisiform. J Hand Surg Am 1985;10:703–7.

22. Rietberg NT, Brown MS, Haase SC. Pisotriquetral pain treated with bilateral pisiform excision in a collegiate diver. J Wrist Surg 2018;7:415–8.

23. Zancolli EA. Medial piso-triquetral instability. Kleinert Institute; 1996. p. XXV.

24. Zancolli EA. Annual meeting Argentine asociation for surgery of the hand 1996.

25. Zancolli ER III. Medial piso-triquetral instability. Budapest, Hungary: Congress Abstracts 9th Congress IFSSH; 2004.

26. Rayan GH. Pisiform ligament complex syndrome and pisotriquetral arthrosis. Hand Clin 2005;21:507–17.

27. Rayan G, Jameson BH, Chung K. The pisotriquetral joint: anatomical, biomechanical and radiographic analysis. J Hand Surg Am 2005;30:596–602.

28. Gardner-Thorpe D, Giddins GEB. A reliable technique for radiographic imaging of the pisotriquetral joint. J Hand Surg Br 1999;24:252.

29. Jameson BH, Rayan GM, Acker RE. radiographic analysis of pisotriquetral joint and pisiform motion. J Hand Surg Am 2002;27:863–9.

Slight Elongation of the Scaphoid and Cancellous Bone Graft Without Compression for Treatment of Scaphoid Nonunions

Igor Golubev, MD

KEYWORDS

- Scaphoid • Nonunion • Arthroscopy • Elongation of scaphoid

KEY POINTS

- In treating scaphoid nonunion, we advocate bone graft with slight scaphoid lengthening.
- We also advocate stabilization of the construct with K-wires without compression.
- Bony union was achieved in the majority of patients as demonstrated in the CT scan.
- Although contrary to contemporary thinking, we consider there are clear benefits to this approach.

INTRODUCTION

Scaphoid nonunion disrupt normal biomechanics of carpus and may result in scaphoid nonunion advanced collapse (SNAC).[1–3] Treatment of scaphoid nonunion includes different types of osteosynthesis with or without correction of deformity[4] and bone grafting.[5] In osteosynthesis of the scaphoid fractures, most authors advocate compression of the construct typically with a headless compression screw.[6–8] Compression will shorten the scaphoid unless already slightly lengthened with bone grafting.

Recently doubts have been raised about the need of compression across scaphoid bone grafting.[9] Some surgeons believe that "natural" bone contact is enough for the union. Options of fixation of scaphoid nonunion include compression screws, K-wires, and plates and screws.[4,10] Among these methods, only screws or plates and screws generate some compression at the zone of nonunion.

BONE GRAFTING IN SCAPHOID NONUNIONS

The role of the bone graft is to bridge the scaphoid gap and to help the bone fragments to unite. The aim of surgery is to restore the structural integrity of the scaphoid to restore reasonably pain-free wrist motion and strength and to avoid long-term symptomatic arthritis. Our preferred method is arthroscopic bone grafting aiming to slightly increase the scaphoid length and stabilize the grafted bone and scaphoid with K-wires. The compressive screws generally have two aims. The first is to bring the bone fragments closer and add compression, which are unnecessary in my opinion. The second is to avoid the rotational mobility of fracture fragments; two or three K-wires can achieve this goal.

Our Surgical Technique

Under brachial plexus block with a standard arthroscopy set-up using 5 kg traction, we routinely only use midcarpal portals for insertion of the arthroscope and probes. Arthroscopic examination starts from the ulnar midcarpal (MCU) portal with a 1.9 or 2.4 mm arthroscope depending on the size of the wrist. The site of the nonunion is defined by the insertion of 18-gauge needle in the joint. Based on this, a radial midcarpal (MCR) or scapho-trapezio-trapezoid (STT) portal created. In the majority, an MCR portal is preferred. We

National Medical Research Center of Traumatology and Orthopedics Named After N.N. Priorov, Moscow, Russia
E-mail address: iog305@mail.ru

Hand Clin 38 (2022) 351–356
https://doi.org/10.1016/j.hcl.2022.04.002
0749-0712/22/© 2022 Elsevier Inc. All rights reserved.

only use the STT portal for nonunion in the distal scaphoid.

Having used both dry and wet arthroscopy, we prefer the dry technique. We find it allows better visualization of the tissues and avoids soft tissue swelling and floating of bone fragments and grafts. The nonunion site is examined with a probe to assess the mobility and density of the fragments and the plane of the nonunion. Bone resection is required in all the cases. We prefer manual bone removal with a small curette and a 2.5 mm bone grasper. In the vast majority of cases, avascular bone and fibrous tissue are easily resected manually. Manual resection also allows for better control of when is enough guided by the presence of bleeding in both fragments. Standard arthroscopic magnification allows the surgeon to see even very small areas of bone bleeding; this is not prevented by the use of a tourniquet as exsanguination will not expel all the blood from the bone. If dorsal mobilization of the distal fragment from fibrotic tissue required, it can be released by use of a soft tissue shaver. We only use an electric burr in rare cases of severe bone sclerosis of one or both fragments. We try to preserve the cartilage of the fragments, but if the underlying bone does not look viable, it needs to be resected with its overlying cartilage.

Once resection is completed to bleeding bone ends, three 1.25 mm K-wires are inserted retrograde under arthroscopic control into the distal fragment. The K-wires are deliberately not placed parallel or close to each other. Each K-wire is passed proximally onto the proximal pole, and its entry into the proximal fragment is assessed. After that, the K-wires are backed out from the proximal fragment, leaving them in the distal pole. The arthroscope is changed from the MCU to the MCR (or STT) portal. The arthroscope is advanced until it is alongside the palmar surface of the scaphoid fossa of the distal radius. The site of the maximum light on the volar radial surface of the distal forearm is marked (**Fig. 1**). We find this point is always on a line between the flexor carpi radialis (FCR) tendon and the radial artery. The camera is moved slightly back dorsally, and a 21G needle is inserted from the marked volar point to the volar intrafragmental space. The position of the needle is controlled by looking at the tip of the needle from inside the wrist. A 4 mm longitudinal incision is made at the needle insertion point and a small straight Mosquito (hemostat) forceps is introduced into the joint by blunt dissection and inserted between the fracture fragments with the tips of the forceps at least 3 mm into the nonunion cavity. The forceps are opened maximally pushing the nonunion fragments apart (**Fig. 2**).

Holding the distracted position, the three K-wires are passed into the proximal fragment,

after which the forceps is removed. On fluoroscopy, the length of the scaphoid, the correction of any dorsal intercalated segment instability (DISI), and the position of the K-wires are assessed (**Fig. 3**). If needed, the manipulation can be repeated after first removing the K-wires from the proximal fragment. The length of the scaphoid, correction of radiolunate angle, and Gilula's arcs are assessed in comparison with radiographs of the contralateral wrist. The gap between the fragments is measured with probes and hooks of a known size to assess how much bone graft is required. In all cases, there is no intrafragmental bone contact, that is, the fragment have been separated completely. The volume of bone graft required is roughly twice what we used to use before performing maximal scaphoid lengthening.

We take cancellous bone graft from the iliac crest. Bone graft is cut into chips not bigger than 3 mm in length/width/depth using a small rongeur. To deliver the bone graft to the scaphoid inside the joint, we use part of an ordinary infusion tube (4 cm long) with one end cut obliquely (**Fig. 4**). The grafted bone is inserted loosely into the infusion tube to deliver to the site of fracture. A nonrigid fragment of the infusion line is introduced into the MCR portal by it oblique end by rotational movements with minimal pressure to reduce soft tissue damage. Under the visual control, the bone is delivered through the infusion line with a slightly smaller trocar with a flat end like the handle of the arthroscopy probe. The nonunion gap is completely filling incrementally by the graft, taking care to fill all the space around and between K-wires. The graft is slightly impacted by applying pressure with a small spatula. Once the construct is checked for stability and avoiding bone impingement against the other carpal bones, the K-wires are cut subcutaneously.

Postoperative Care

The wrist is immobilized in a short arm cast for 8 weeks when a wrist computed tomography (CT) is performed to check for the bone union. If there are clear signs of bone union, the K-wires are removed in an operating theater under local anesthetic, and rehabilitation started. In doubt, a new short-arm plaster cast is applied and the CT scan repeated at 12 weeks when the K wires are removed (**Fig. 5**). If there is still doubt, the plaster cast is kept on beyond 12 weeks.

OUR PATIENTS AND CLINICAL RESULTS

From 2014 to 2020, we operated upon 134 patients (134 scaphoid fractures) for scaphoid nonunion. The first 64 patients were treated

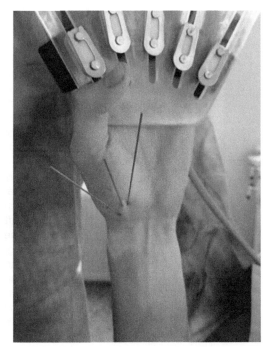

Fig. 1. Light at the volar wrist surface showing the palmar projection of nonunion.

without lengthening using the Linscheid maneuver (correction of the extended position of the proximal pole of the scaphoid and lunate by flexing the wrist to realign the extended lunate with the radius), but we found the scaphoid was often not restored to its normal length. Of these 31 (48%) had complete follow-up (clinical examination, radiographs, and CT scans); 14 had only X-ray follow-up and 19 were lost to follow-up. 26 of the 31 (84%) scaphoids achieved bone union on CT scans. Among the 14 scaphoids assessed only

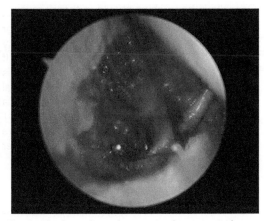

Fig. 2. The branches of mosquito hemostatic forceps are maximally opened pushing the fragments apart.

with radiographs, 10 had some sign of union and 4 scaphoids were found to have nonunion. Overall, 36 of 45 (80%) with radiographic follow-up of some degree had clear evidence of bone union.

We performed the new technique of scaphoid lengthening in 70 patients (70 wrists). Correction of the DISI was achieved in all these patients. 42 patients had completely follow-up (clinical examination, radiographs, and CT scans). 41 of 42 (98%) achieved bone union. Of the 17 with radiographic follow-up alone, 9 achieved bone union but in 8 we could not be sure; 11 were lost to follow-up. Overall, 50 of 59 (85%) with radiographic follow-up of some degree had clear evidence of bone union.

The mean DASH and VAS pain scores and ranges of wrist motion improved in both series, but the patients in the later series had better recovery of their radio-scaphoid angles.

CONSIDERATIONS AND IMPLICATIONS
Limitations

We had quite a high loss to follow-up not least because the patients moved away or did not want to be followed up. This is very common in our institute and our country. The high rate of loss to follow-up makes an assessment of the rate of union less reliable. However, based on the patients who had been followed up and examined with CT scan, the union rate is very high; over 80% overall, and 98% in the later series when we attempted to "elongate" the scaphoid. Although we cannot make firm conclusions based on the patient series with a high loss of follow-up, our findings encourage us that lengthening the scaphoid in treating nonunion with bone graft may be of importance. In addition, because we used K-wire fixation without compression in all these patients, we also argue that compression may be less necessary than current mainstream belief and practice suggest.

In scaphoid nonunion, angulation and shortening of the scaphoid always occur.[11–13] Arthroscopic surgical correction protects most of the soft tissue structures and vascular anatomy of the wrist.[9] Magnification at arthroscopy makes bone resection precise and theoretically less traumatic.

Compression across bone unions is recommended in the majority of textbooks and often is considered necessary after bone grafts. However, bone distraction may also positively influence bone regeneration.[14] Fixation of scaphoid nonunion without compression may not influence the rate of bone union.[15–20]

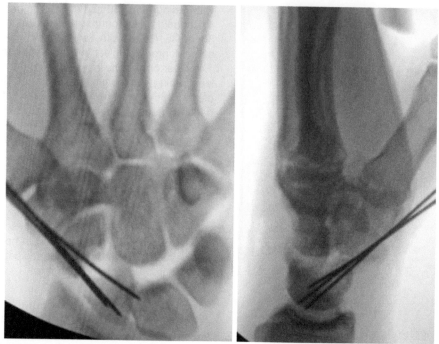

Fig. 3. After fixation, the length of the scaphoid, the degree of DISI correction, the reposition of the fragments, and the position of the K-wire were assessed.

Cancellous Bone Grafting (Without Compression) May be a Better Treatment for Scaphoid Nonunion than Cortico-cancellous Bone Grafting

Nonunion of scaphoid waist fractures often involves dorsal apex angulation with bone loss and collapse. The standard treatment of scaphoid waist nonunion with bone loss is structural cortico-cancellous bone grafting with internal fixation.[21] Cancellous bone graft also has been used to treat unstable scaphoid nonunion with good results.[22] When K-wire fixation was used without any compression of the grafted bone, we achieved bony union in 30 of 34 patients (88%).[22]

Comparison of outcomes between cortico-cancellous bone graft and cancellous bone graft demonstrates that the cancellous bone graft with rigid fixation led to earlier bony union than the cortico-cancellous bone graft. In addition, cancellous bone graft showed similar restoration of alignment and no difference has been shown in wrist functional outcomes between the two methods.[23] Cancellous bone graft appears to give earlier bone union and can be used in a minimally invasive fashion.[9] We consider that cancellous bone is superior to cortico-cancellous one. However, one key technical point is not to compress the grafted cancellous bone, which is not often stressed by many authors. In contrast, compression to the grafted cancellous bone is very often seen in clinical practice.

Cancellous bone chips should in theory revascularize more quickly and reliably than a solid cortico-cancellous bone graft. This is another theoretic advantage especially if compression across these nonunion is not required.

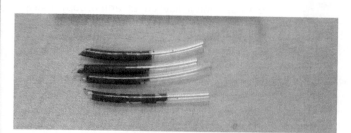

Fig. 4. For bone graft insertion, 4-cm long fragments of infusion line cutting in the oblique plane were used.

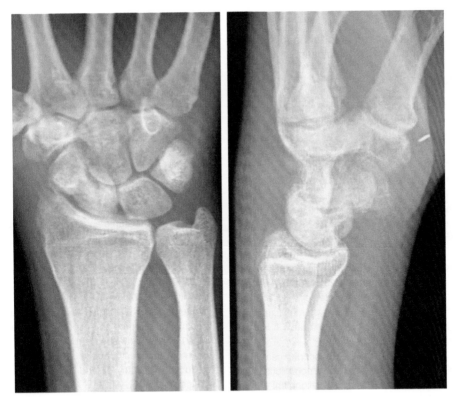

Fig. 5. Bone union in 12 weeks after the procedure.

An Arthroscopic Approach Can Lengthen the Scaphoid with Bone Grafting

Can we correct scaphoid deformity arthroscopically? The answer is "Yes." In performing arthroscopic bone grafting, distal fragment joystick manipulation is not so effective as the main deformity is in the proximal fragment. An additional volar portal with direct correction of the deformity is more effective, safe, and predictable in our hands.

As shown in our patients, this approach is practical and has led to a high union rate. In the patients with bone grafting and slight lengthening of the scaphoid with bone graft, the healing rate is even higher. Slight overcorrection of scaphoid length, which is possible using direct pressure on the nonunion fragments, allows correction of any DISI deformity.[24] It restores natural ligamentous/carpal balance, which also helps to contain the bone graft in the correct place. Slight overcorrection also allows correction of the typical (but often not appreciated) protonation and dorsal subluxation of the distal scaphoid fragment, which is often hard to correct, without open mobilization. In our experience, elongation of the scaphoid nonunion corrects the protonation and subluxation of the distal nonunion fragment secondary to pressure on the STT joint, which reduces the distal fragment to its correct position.

SUMMARY

In summary, based on the results of our patients, we advocate slight lengthening of the scaphoid with cancellous bone grafting and K-wire stabilization while acknowledging there are limitations in our study especially the number of patients with no or incomplete follow-up.

CLINICS CARE POINTS

- In treating scaphoid nonunion, we advocate bone graft with slight scaphoid lengthening.
- We also advocate stabilization of the construct with K-wires without compression.
- Bony union was achieved in the majority of patients as demonstrated in the CT scan.

ACKNOWLEDGMENTS

Grigory Balyura, MD, contributed to the follow-up of the patients and functional evaluation.

REFERENCES

1. Gehrmann S, Roeger T, Kaufmann R, et al. Wrist motion analysis in scaphoid nonunion. Eur J Trauma Emerg Surg 2016;42:11–4.

2. Moritomo H, Murase T, Oka K, et al. Relationship between the fracture location and the kinematic pattern in scaphoid nonunion. J Hand Surg Am 2008;33:1459–68.

3. Waitayawinyu T, McCallister WV, Nemechek NM, et al. Scaphoid nonunion. J Am Acad Orthop Surg 2007;15:308–20.

4. Pinder RM, Brkljac M, Rix L, et al. Treatment of scaphoid nonunion: a systematic review of the existing evidence. J Hand Surg Am 2015;40:1797–805.

5. Ferguson DO, Shanbhag V, Hedley H, et al. Scaphoid fracture non-union: a systematic review of surgical treatment using bone graft. J Hand Surg Eur 2016;41:492–500.

6. Kim JP, Seo JB, Yoo JY, et al. Arthroscopic management of chronic unstable scaphoid nonunions: effects on restoration of carpal alignment and recovery of wrist function. Arthroscopy 2015;31:460–9.

7. Zemirline A, Lebailly F, Taleb C, et al. Arthroscopic treatment of scaphoid nonunion with humpback deformity and DISI with corticocancellous bone grafting: Technical note. Hand Surg Rehabil 2019;38:280–5.

8. Hegazy G. Percutaneous screw fixation of scaphoid waist fracture non-union without bone grafting. J Hand Microsurg 2015;7:250–5.

9. Clara Wong WY, Ho PC. Arthroscopic management of scaphoid nonunion. Hand Clin 2019;35:295–313.

10. Eng K, Gill S, Hoy S, et al. Volar scaphoid plating for nonunion: a multicenter case series study. J Wrist Surg 2020;9:225–9.

11. Gillette BP, Amadio PC, Kakar S. Long-term outcomes of scaphoid malunion. Hand 2017;12:26–30.

12. Lee CH, Lee KH, Kim DY, et al. Clinical outcome of scaphoid malunion as a result of scaphoid fracture nonunion surgical treatment: a 5-year minimum follow-up study. Orthop Traumatol Surg Res 2015;101:359–63.

13. Mathoulin CL, Arianni M. Treatment of the scaphoid humpback deformity - is correction of the dorsal intercalated segment instability deformity critical? J Hand Surg Eur 2018;43:13–23.

14. Kim UK, Chung IK, Lee KH, et al. Bone regeneration in mandibular distraction osteogenesis combined with compression stimulation. J Oral Maxillofac Surg 2006;64:1498–505.

15. Hegazy G, Seddik M, Abd-Elghany T, et al. Treatment of unstable scaphoid waist nonunion with cancellous bone grafts and cannulated screw or Kirschner wire fixation. J Plast Surg Hand Surg 2021;55:167–72.

16. Fernandez DL. The Author's technique for the management of unstable scaphoid nonunions: tips and tricks. Hand Clin 2019;35:271–9.

17. Yeo JH, Kim JY. Surgical strategy for scaphoid nonunion treatment. J Hand Surg Asian Pac 2018;23:450–62.

18. Schweizer A, Mauler F, Vlachopoulos L, et al. Computer-assisted 3 dimensional reconstructions of scaphoid fractures and nonunions with and without the use of patient-specific guides: early clinical outcomes and postoperative assessments of reconstruction accuracy. J Hand Surg Am 2016;41:59–69.

19. Giusti G, Bishop AT, Shin AY. Overstuffing of unstable scaphoid nonunions: a radiographic analysis of carpal parameters. J Hand Surg Am 2019;44:423.e1–6.

20. Capito AE, Higgins JP. Scaphoid overstuffing: the effects of the dimensions of scaphoid reconstruction on scapholunate alignment. J Hand Surg Am 2013;38:2419–25.

21. Sayegh ET, Strauch RJ. Graft choice in the management of unstable scaphoid nonunion: a systematic review. J Hand Surg Am 2014;39:1500–6.

22. Park HY, Yoon JO, Jeon IH, et al. A comparison of the rates of union after cancellous iliac crest bone graft and Kirschner-wire fixation in the treatment of stable and unstable scaphoid nonunion. Bone Joint J 2013;95-B:809–14.

23. Kim JK, Yoon JO, Baek H. Corticocancellous bone graft vs cancellous bone graft for the management of unstable scaphoid nonunion. Orthop Traumatol Surg Res 2018;104:115–20.

24. Furey MJ, White NJ, Dhaliwal GS. Scapholunate ligament injury and the effect of scaphoid lengthening. J Wrist Surg 2020;9:76–80.

10 Hypotheses in Hand Surgery

Jin Bo Tang, MD

KEYWORDS

- Hypothesis • Peripheral nerve compression • Double crush of the nerve • Early active motion
- Hand elevation

KEY POINTS

- Neuritis of the anterior interosseous nerve (AIN) exists, but entrapment of this nerve does not.
- When a nerve is entrapped proximally, its distal part becomes swollen and often compressed by normal structures. The "double crush" by entrapment at two levels is less common.
- Starting motion therapy of the hand within a week after surgery can be replaced with starting motion therapy at 2 or 3 weeks in most patients.
- Short splints will be used more frequently in the future.
- Proximal pole fractures of the scaphoid should be conservatively treated more frequently.
- Elevation of the operated hand after surgery is unnecessary unless the trauma or surgery is extensive or severe hand edema is expected.

INTRODUCTION

I have assembled several hypotheses because answers for these topics are unclear or unproven. Some are my preferred approaches, but I have found no proof whether they are better than the alternative methods used by others. Therefore, I present them for interested colleagues to prove or disprove them. Collective publication of the hypotheses may also stimulate thinking, clinical observation, and highlight several areas of possible research interest.

When there is no solid evidence to support superiority of one treatment method over another, we have to decide which method to use. If the method leads to expected results in our own patients, we tend to continue to use it. The continuation of the personal proffered approaches is largely based on good outcomes of our own patients and on faith. The practices that I continue to use have led to expected results in my patients, but some were in small numbers, which are of exploratory nature; and it is possible that the other methods lead to better outcomes.

I present the thoughts and practices of several disorders in the form of *hypotheses* to reflect the lack of good proof or certainties and call attention to questions that they raise. Proving or disproving these hypotheses may enhance understandings or treatment of these disorders, improve patient outcomes, or reduce discomfort of the patients. I hope that colleagues consider these hypotheses and collect evidence to support or disapprove them.

HYPOTHESIS 1
Neuritis of the Anterior Interosseous Nerve Exists, but Entrapment Does Not

I put this as the first hypothesis because this topic was recently discussed among several senior surgeons,[1–4] and the consensus was that anterior interosseous nerve (AIN) entrapment may not exist. It is possible that the swollen AIN after neuritis initiates compression by the normal structures that surround it (**Fig. 1**). Immediate decompression of the AIN may eliminate such compression, and symptoms can disappear

Department of Hand Surgery, Affiliated Hospital of Nantong University, 20 West Temple Road, Nantong 226001, Jiangsu, China
E-mail address: jinbotang@yahoo.com

Hand Clin 38 (2022) 357–366
https://doi.org/10.1016/j.hcl.2022.04.003
0749-0712/22/© 2022 Elsevier Inc. All rights reserved.

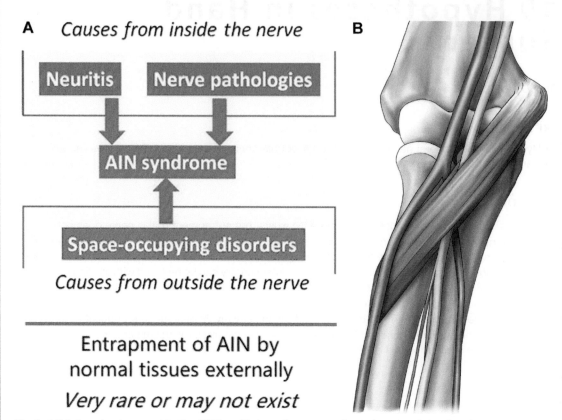

A *Causes from inside the nerve*

Neuritis   Nerve pathologies

AIN syndrome

Space-occupying disorders

Causes from outside the nerve

Entrapment of AIN by
normal tissues externally
Very rare or may not exist

B

Fig. 1. (*A*) External entrapment to the AIN is unlikely and may not exist as the nerve is small and tissues around it are soft. Neuritis causes swollen nerve to be compressed by surrounding normal tissues, leading to AIN palsy. (*B*) Anatomical location of the AIN. (copyright Julia Ruston).

immediately; but without surgical decompression, the symptoms may spontaneously subside after weeks or months. The question remains whether immediate surgical decompression without lengthy conservative treatment is worthwhile.

The AIN is a very small nerve. There is no hard tissues around it. It is very unlikely to be compressed if the nerve itself is normal. However, if neuritis exists, this small swollen nerve may sustain compression from surrounding normal tissues. The clinical symptoms and signs of AIN palsy are caused by the swollen nerve, which would spontaneously recover once swelling goes down without the need of surgical decompression of the normal tissue around this nerve.

Based on what we know, it is better to consider that AIN entrapment *by the normal tissues* surrounding it does not exist. I have not read any definite writings on the existence of AIN entrapment neuropathy. Such entrapment is merely a hypothesis and may not exist at all. Neuropathy inside the AIN, such as hour-glass constriction, is *nerve* pathology and does not involve entrapment.

HYPOTHESIS 2
When a Nerve Is Entrapped Proximally, Distally It Becomes Swollen and Often Compressed by Normal Structures. Mechanical Entrapment at Two Levels Is less Common

There are a lot of uncertainties and disagreements regarding double crush syndrome. This term was first used in 1973, after Upton and McComas[5] had assessed a large group of patients with cervical root lesions and upper extremity peripheral entrapment neuropathies—either carpal tunnel syndrome (CTS), ulnar neuropathy at the elbow, or both. They proposed that focal compression often occurs at more than one level along the course of a single nerve fiber.

Upton and McComas[5] proposed that under these circumstances, a disturbance of axonal transport caused by compression at the proximal site, for example, the cervical root, may impair the capacity of the nerve segment distal to it to resist further focal compressive injury. Consequently, an otherwise subclinical focal entrapment neuropathy (eg, CTS) could convert into a clinically evident one. They theorized that asymptomatic compression at one site predisposed a nerve to increased susceptibility to impairment at a distal site.[5] Upton and McComas[5] further assumed that this may occur even though the proximal lesion, although symptomatic, was not clinically severe. Therefore, a cervical radiculopathy presenting as little more than neck pain and stiffness could still precipitate a distal focal entrapment neuropathy. Neural ischemia, inherent elastic characteristics of the nerve, and systemic conditions such as diabetes and thyroid disease render the nerve's distal segment prone to compression by normal tissues surrounding it.

I agree with these analyses and observations. Therefore, the need for decompression at two sites is only a hypothesis. If the proximal mechanical entrapment is released, the distal part of this nerve is likely no longer compressed by normal tissues over time. The current suggestion and practice of releasing two sites of a doubly crushed nerve is therefore unnecessary. In discussing treatment, it is important to note the difference between "compression" and "entrapment"; the latter indicates constriction by hard, often pathologic, structures external to the nerve.

The double crush syndrome is debated because (1) there is no way to objectively ascertain that symptoms ascribed to this syndrome are the result of pathophysiology at two levels of a peripheral nerve; (2) this speculative pathophysiology is applied when patients have more symptoms, disability, or dissatisfaction than expected; and (3) the concept of double crush may encourage additional surgery at another level when surgery may not be necessary or the most effective treatment option.[6–10] These debates further add to my arguments that the compression to the distal part of the nerve may not necessarily need surgical intervention.

However, it is much less certain that compression can occur at two sites by *external mechanical entrapment* of a nerve. Osterman[11] found that given a more proximal root compression, less compression of the median nerve in the carpal tunnel was required to produce symptoms. He found that 90% of patients with concomitant cervical radiculopathy had proximal radiation of pain compared with 50% of patients with CTS alone. He noted that fewer than half the patients with concomitant cervical radiculopathy had median nerve paresthesia, compared with 93% of patients with CTS alone. The results indicate distinctive differences between double crush syndrome, which presents with CTS, and isolated CTS. Although patients with compression of the cervical nerve roots commonly have symptoms in upper extremity, most of these patients do not have mechanical entrapment distally.[12–14]

External mechanical entrapment of a nerve at two distinct sites, such as one proximal in the cervical spine, and the other distal in the cubital tunnel, carpal tunnel, or elsewhere, is uncommon or rare, although possible. The nerve trunk, which is entraped at two sites, both distal to the cervical spine, may be even more uncommon (**Fig. 2**).

I suggest that when the cervical spine has definite signs of degeneration, the treatment of the distal compression site should be considered cautiously, especially when nerve compression at a distal site is suspected in the proximal forearm, such as for radial tunnel syndrome or FDS-pronator syndrome. The compression at these sites may be secondary, and release of these sites may improve but not completely restore the strength of the affected muscles.

Many spine surgeons who diagnose cervical radiculopathy do not routinely look for any specific sites of compression in forearm. Similarly hand surgeons who diagnose the compression of nerve in forearm do not usually make a diagnosis of cervical radiculopathy. It is likely that if the spine surgeons looked at the forearm to check any potential sites of compression, they would found these secondary compression sites (I called it secondary, because the nerve may be swollen and compressed by normal tissues around it). On the contrary, some hand surgeons, who commonly examine the forearm without routinely checking the status of cervical spine, may find compression in the forearm and consider these patients have the forearm entrapment neuropathy as the initiating sites of compression. In these patients, decompression at the forearm would lead to immediate relief of compression and restoration of muscle function, but recovery may not be complete because of primary compression site is in the cervical spine.

Therefore, is there a merit in decompressing the distal (secondary) compression site along a nerve trunk when the cervical spine is definitely compressing the nerve roots?

There are two hypotheses regarding the treatment. If the decompression at the distal site would greatly relieve the symptoms, this surgery should be advocated. This will hugely increase the number of surgical cases in patients with cervical nerve root compression. But, it is also plausible that the decompression at the distal site is not necessary, because over a certain period of time, the symptoms may subside spontaneously, or the symptoms may recur after temporary relief following the surgical decompression at the distal site. I wish future investigations would prove or disprove this quandary.

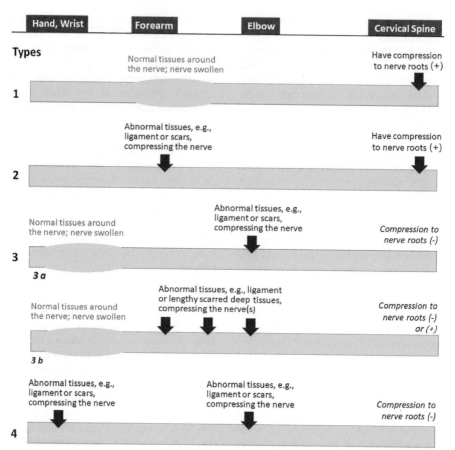

Fig. 2. My classification and thoughts on four types of double and multiple crush at a nerve trunk. I consider a regional pain syndrome is multiple crush to nerves (see type 3b). Therefore this syndrome does not need a specific term. Multiple crush offer explain to this condition. Type 1: entrapment of a given nerve occurs at cervical spine with swollen nerve compressed at another distal site in the upper extremity. Type 2: entrapment at cervical spine and another distal site caused by abnormal tissues outside the nerve occur, which is quite commonly seen. The incidence may be lower than Type 1. Type 3: Along a given nerve trunk, one entrapment at a proximal site and compression at a distal site because the distal nerve segment is swollen, which is more easily compressed by normal ligaments. This type is further divided to 3a, in which compression occurs at only two sites, and 3b, in which compression occurs at multiple sites, as seen in conditions of severe deep tissue scarring after multiple surgeries or severe trauma. This condition can occur with or without compression at the cervical spine level. Type 3b is a condition of complex pain syndrome, which I consider it multiple crush to the nerves in and beyond the area of scars. Type 4, entrapment at two sites caused by abnormal tissues outside the nerve, which may or may not exist. Type 1 is the most common, for which the need of decompression at the distal compression site may favor faster recovery, but its value is not well defined, and further studies are needed. Other types are less common with the similar questions for the need and timing of surgery.

The upper extremity with multiple surgeries or severe trauma would create extensive scar, which will produce multiple constriction sites to the nerves in the elbow, forearm or wrist, depending on the sites of surgery or trauma. I tend to expand neurological pain after these conditions with a term multiple crush syndrome. This is my expanded term after double crush. The multiple crush can be the causes of currently called condition of complex regional pain syndrome. This condition is only a more severe or extreme form of nerve compression by scarred tissues in a lengthy area. I personally use small surgical incisions and I am very careful in surgical dissection. I do not see such patients after my operations, but I did see a few who had very severe trauma to the forearm. Therefore, release of the scarred deep tissues in the area of trauma is in fact a decompression surgery to the nerves. Decompression of the nerves distal to the area of scar may also benefit recovery of nerve function distal to the decompression site because the nerve segment distal to the area of severely scarred deep tissues is often swollen and subjected to secondary compression more easily. Such decompression surgery would decrease pain and improve hand function. This is a multiple crush condition extending to the distal normal areas, when the proximal scarred deep tissues are lengthy and the nerves distal to the site are more easily compressed by normal tissues, e.g., ligaments (Type 3 in **Fig. 2**).

HYPOTHESIS 3
Early Surgical Decompression to Forearm Entrapment Neuropathy Is Beneficial to Help Speedy Recovery and Avoid Symptoms and Dysfunction Associated with Lengthy Conservative Treatment

Continuing with the discussion in hypothesis 2, this hypothesis is not about long-term outcome but rather the possible merits of immediate relief of symptoms with surgical intervention.

I have discussed this with a surgeon who operated a lot of patients with median and radial nerve compressions in the proximal forearm. I agree that early surgical release without commonly suggested lengthy conservative treatment (6 months) may have merits. The immediate return of the muscle powers of the fingers and thumb in proximal median nerve compression, or relief of the symptoms of patients with radial tunnel syndrome, means that patients does not need to endure months of symptoms. If immediate relief is possible, the surgeries appear worthy. This is even true the surgery is through a small incision and less invasive.

Nevertheless a few concerns need clarification. (1) If the surgeries are done at initial clinical visits without more than 6 months of observation, do the symptoms and strength return to normal, or is there only partial recovery? Immediate and complete recovery of the muscle strength during surgery or right after surgery could be the results of local anesthesia plus surgical decompression, which is not equal to longterm relief or recovery. (2) There should be a control cohort of patients, who do not have surgical release and who are followed for a length comparable to the patients with early surgical decompression, to address the possibility of natural recovery. Immediate return of function following surgery cannot address these concerns. Early surgical decompression may not be worthwhile if its functional recovery is insufficient or if there is similar recovery without surgery.

These questions need to be addressed through clinical studies to establish the exact value of early surgical decompression although an immediate relief of the problems will reduce the suffering of these patients for months when observation is used.

Such early surgical decompression may be used for a subset of the patients who can gladly afford the surgery and are happy to have the surgery to gain fast relief and fast return to job. I guess the early surgical intervention is helpful although often unnecessary. Therefore, the early surgery is justified only in the patients who wish to skip several month of continuing symptoms in the conservative treatment. However, this may not be the preference of many other patients with surgical cost and risk taken into consideration. The patient has to be informed about the possibility of recovery without the early surgical decompression and about the risks of surgery. If surgery is decided, the surgeons should always make a precise diagnosis about the site of compression and use a small surgical incision to make the surgery less invasive.[15,16]

HYPOTHESIS 4
Ruptured Digital Flexor Tendons Can Be Repaired Directly After a Quite Lengthy Delay, and Muscle Elasticity Can Be Restored

Several surgeons have already voice this possibility, but clinical data are insufficient to define exact length of delay and in what circumstances this delayed primary repair is possible and should be attempted. I do not have a large number of the patients who came to me a month after trauma. I found in several of them, however, that I could do primary repairs, even after 3 or 6 months, and they finally recovered digital function without additional surgery. Questions remain regarding how long is "quite lengthy". I regularly perform delayed primary repairs in patients coming to me within 4 weeks after clean-cut injuries. Because the area of scar is limited, I excise the scar and fibrotic pulleys. Most of the pulleys are intact, and none need reconstruction. A direct end-to-end tendon repair is possible.

When a patient presents 4–6 weeks after trauma, a primary repair, although with some difficulty, may still be worthy in most patients. After week 6, a decision to perform a direct repair is made according to intraoperative findings. In some, direct repair is possible. Which is better after a lengthy delay, delayed primary repair or secondary tendon grafting? The answer is unknown.

Another hypothesis is that muscle elasticity is restored even after months of delay, and given lengthy rehabilitation, the fingers with delayed tendon repairs will be fully extendable and function well. There is such a case report of recovery of muscle elasticity.[17] Lengthening of the tendons in the forearm is another solution if muscle elasticity does not recover.[18] For delayed direct repair, rehabilitation will need to last longer,

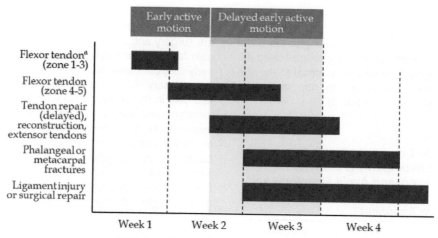

Fig. 3. The ranges of starting the partial-range active flexion of the finger or thumb are indicated with ruby red bars, which differ in each disorder. The exact timing is decided within the timeframes with consideration of situations of individual patients and the structures repaired. [a]Not include zone 1A, where no motion over the first two weeks after surgery.

and patients should be compliant. When the tendon is impossible to be pulled together under tension in attempted delayed direct repair, surgeon should considerarvesting a tendon graft to replace the lacerated tendon 3 months after initial trauma.

HYPOTHESIS 5
Starting Motion Therapy Within a Week after Surgery Can Be Delayed to Week 2 or 3 in Most Patients

In my practice, except for primary flexor tendon repair, I do not start "immediate" early active motion, and this practice has served me well.[19] I usually start motion therapy at week 2 to 3 depending on structures repaired or surgeries done (**Fig. 3**). I have not found any major problems with delaying the initiation of motion therapy. I learnt other surgeons to start early active motion from very first week after surgery and have doubted whether this is necessary or makes much difference from the "delayed" early active motion.

I have attempted to find evidence of the superiority of one method over the other and have not found any, perhaps because delayed early active motion is not commonly prescribed. A comparison of immediate early motion therapy and delayed early motion therapy has not been done. If delayed early active motion produces equal or similar outcomes without increasing the incidence of finger or hand stiffness months after surgery, a delay would decrease the patient's pain, the risk of fracture displacement (if internal fixation of the fracture

is done), and the risk of rupturing the repaired tissues (such as collateral ligaments, extensor tendons). I will continue to adopt delayed early active motion and wait to see whether investigators reveal whether there are remarkable differences according to when active motion therapy starts. My hypothesis is that early and delayed early motion have equal outcomes weeks and months after surgery.

HYPOTHESIS 6
Short Splints Will Be Used in Many More Patients in the Years to Come

I see the use of a short splint a future trend as we understand more and more about tissue healing and we improve the mechanical strength of surgical repairs. After flexor tendon repair, a short splint (from wrist to fingertip or from forearm to fingertip) is already popular.[20–22] After extensor tendon repair in the fingers or thumb, a shorter splint from distal forearm to the digital tip is fine, because the currently used surgical repair methods are strong, which can tolerate a lot of tension in the tendon.

For the treatment of hand fractures (excluding scaphoid fracture), metacarpal fractures can be treated with a short splint from wrist to the palm or with a short splint in the palm as shown in a recent report.[23] If the surgeon prefers more protection, a splint from the distal forearm to the proximal phalanx level is sufficient. Also for the finger fractures, a short splint is sufficient. A general principle is that the splint only needs to span one joint

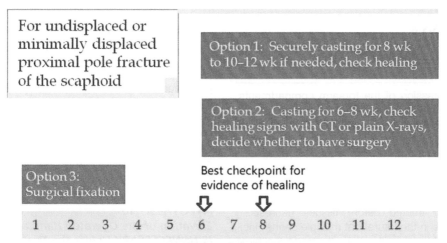

For undisplaced or minimally displaced proximal pole fracture of the scaphoid

Option 1: Securely casting for 8 wk to 10–12 wk if needed, check healing

Option 2: Casting for 6–8 wk, check healing signs with CT or plain X-rays, decide whether to have surgery

Option 3: Surgical fixation

Best checkpoint for evidence of healing

1 2 3 4 5 6 7 8 9 10 11 12

Weeks after fracture

Fig. 4. Summary of currently equally valid treatment options for nondisplaced or minimally displaced proximal pole fracture of the scaphoid. The proximal pole is defined as proximal 20% of the scaphoid. Each option have support of clinical data and reasons. The clinical decision can be variable depending on patient's wishes, economic burden of the surgery, and also surgeon's own judgment of these reasons and data. I should stress the cast should be secure and firm when options 1 and 2 are chosen, and options 1 and 2 are not inferior options. The week 6 to 8 is the clinical checkpoint for the healing with CT or plain X-rays if option 2 is chosen. The current clinical data do not support any one *against* the others.

distal to the fractured bone and one joint proximal. Unnecessary extension of the distal part of the splint over fingers is extremely harmful, as finger joints are small and prone to stiffness. This general principle is often forgotten by junior surgeons, who are the ones that usually make plaster splints for these patients. I hypothesize that more short splints will be used in hand surgery in the future and wish that colleagues consider them and use more frequently.

HYPOTHESIS 7
Fractures of the Scaphoid Proximal Pole Are Treated Conservatively by Many Surgeons

The proximal pole fracture involves the proximal 20% of the scaphoid and is uncommon (<5% of all scaphoid fractures). Published data on union incidence can lead to different treatment recommendations. The suggestion of using surgical treatment for this fracture is based on reported 20% to 50% (on average 1/3) incidences of nonunion after casting.[24,25] This same healing incidence can also be interpreted as two-third of the cases do not need surgery. A more recent study showed that 90% of 52 undisplaced proximal pole fractures noted on CT healed with cast immobilization.[24]

I have always use casting to treat nondisplaced proximal pole fractures of the scaphoid, and these patients have not needed later surgery (I do see nonunions in patients who have not any

immobilization at all for months, because they did not see a doctor for months after trauma.) I cast these patients with a fresh distal pole fracture first for 7 to 8 weeks. If they are not yet healed (**Fig. 4**), I prolong the casting up to 10 or 12 weeks. I do not recall any patients who failed to heal and needed surgery eventually, although I might have missed follow-up of one or two out of about 20 patients with these fractures in the past 2 decades. For these patients, I make a very secure cast myself for these patients, ensure the cast is not loose over the wrist and padding is not too thick, so the wrist does not move inside the cast. I observed some surgeons or plaster technicians make a very loose cast and padding is thick. I suspect this loose cast will lead to insecure fixation and certainly risk non-union of the scaphoid pole. A below-elbow cast is applied extending distally to the MP joint. Although above observations are not a concrete report of a patient cohort, my experience with my patients and published information do not lead me to surgical fixation for those nondisplaced or minimally displaced fractures. Several other senior surgeons have similar views.[26–28]

I predict that nondisplaced and minimally displaced proximal pole scaphoid fractures will be treated with casting primarily by many hand surgeons in the future. In majority of the patients, internal fixation of the proximal pole fracture may be unnecessary and only invites complications. In making a cast one must attend to casting details and do not make a loose cast.

HYPOTHESIS 8
Compartment Syndrome in the Forearm Is Treated with Multiple Shorter Incisions Without Skin Graft in Most Patients

In decompression of the forearm compartments, classical teaching is a long S-shaped incision, often followed later by a skin graft. This is proper in a severe case of forearm compartment syndrome, which needs extensive debridement of nonviable tissues and thorough decompression of the nerves and vessels. In modern times, such severe involvement is seldom seen, because the patient is diagnosed and treated before tissues necrosis. I hypothesize in the future that multiple shorter incision in the forearm will replace the traditional large incision and not require a skin graft. I decompress 2 to 3 patients yearly on average and have not needed to skin graft them. With 4 to 5 shorter incisions (usually ranging 3–10 cm), skin grafting has not been necessary, because the skin could be closed as swelling came down. A Jacob's ladder with vessel loops can further help with skin closure without skin grafting and decrease the size of scar. I predict that this approach will be recognized more widely and will replace a long incision in most of these patients.

HYPOTHESIS 9
Small Free or Pedicled Flap Transfers to Fingers Will No Longer Be Used as Artificial Skin Substitutes Become Popular

Many of my colleagues find that they use smaller flaps in the hand less frequently in recent years. Even large free flap transfers are less often necessary because of the use of artificial dermal templates for small defects and *vacuum-assisted* closure of a large defect, which stimulates formation of granulation tissue and allows epithelialization over the granulation tissue. I use Integra (*Integra* LifeSciences, Plainsboro, NJ) in patients with defects in dorsal aspect of the finger (including the distal nail defects) and have found that epithelization on the dorsum of the hand occurs easily and functions well. For defects on the volar aspect of the fingers, advancement flaps with or without neurovascular pedicles are sufficient. I have found transfer of small free flaps to the fingers is no longer needed, and even the pedicled small flaps from outside the injured finger may not be needed, as a dermal template can be used instead, and local advancement flaps covering a part of the defect while leaving a 1 to 2 cm of defect for self-regeneration. It seems just a matter of time that most surgeons recognize this approach and use it in most patients.

I hypothesize that small free or pedicled flap transfers to fingers will no longer be necessary as artificial skin substitutes become popular. I see the repair of the soft tissue defects in the fingers become easier and cause less, or no, morbidity in the sites other than the injured finger itself. I have seen such a wonderful shift in my practice, which made it easier for me and patients happier. In fact, sensory recovery of the regenerated tissues with these new approaches is also pleasant.

HYPOTHESIS 10
Elevation of the Operated Hand after Surgery IS UNNECESSARY Unless the Trauma or Surgery Is Extensive or Severe Hand Edema Is Expected

I was brought up in my training and practice to instruct patients to elevate their hands to after major surgery that might cause marked edema of the hand or upper extremity. I encountered colleagues who give postoperative orders to almost all patients to elevate their operated hands, sometimes to the level of the head. I do not see reports that such elevation improves outcomes. It is possible that elevation decreases pain, and indeed sometimes the patient feels more comfortable to elevate the hand to the chest level after surgery, but such elevation does not need to be the case in all or many patients. Raising the hand high is plainly unnecessary. I have not seen any solid evidence. I am sure that elevation over the head or above chest level for days is tiresome for patients. When I have told patients that they do not need to elevate their hand, they feel immediately happier. Any of us would agree elevating a hand to the head level for 30 min causes a lot of discomfort. Therefore I wonder whether hand elevation to head level adds more discomfort to the patient than a localized hand procedure itself.

There is no need to instruct the patients to elevate the hand with minor lacerations, simple fractures, or after minor surgeries in the hand. After surgeries in the fingers or hand—simple pinning of fractures, flexor or extensor tendon repairs, finger joint releases, and so on—I only tell the patients to put the hand where it makes them comfortable and that they may use a sling to secure the hand at or below the chest with the elbow flexed, which prevents the hand from dropping. With this degree of hand elevation, the patients feel very comfortable. Elevation above the chest level is helpful in instances of major tissue disturbances in the hand or and surgeries involving forearm especially the muscles, but the practice does not need to be extended to minor, localized operations.

Should a comparative clinical study be performed, we might find the discomfort caused by elevation of the hand to an uncomfortable position adds to the patients' discomfort. I hypothesize that such unnecessary hand elevation is more widely recognized, and that a large number of patients will benefit from not being advised by the surgeon to assume uncomforting hand positions. In past years, I explained why intrinsic plus position of the hand is almost unnecessary and many colleagues do not use it now.[29] Unnecessary hand elevation may be another source of discomfort, and for a localized and small procedure, its discomfort may overweigh that of the surgery.

SUMMARY

I have put together the several topics and labeled them as hypotheses. My preferred approaches and practices are outlined and the rationales or considerations are given. Some are different from those used by others, but I have found no proof whether my methods are better or worse than those used by others. These hypotheses are to stimulate thinking, clinical observation and investigations, and highlight several areas of future research. I hope clarification will improve our understanding of these topics and thereby avoid unnecessary surgeries and treatments and improve patients' postoperative comfort and long-term outcomes.

CLINICS CARE POINTS

- Neuritis of the anterior interosseous nerve (AIN) exists, but entrapment of this nerve does not.

- When a nerve is entrapped proximally, its distal part becomes swollen and often compressed by normal structures. The "double crush" by entrapment at two levels is less common.

- Starting motion therapy within a week after surgery can be replaced with starting motion therapy at 2 or 3 weeks in most patients. Only the patient with primary flexor tendon repair need initiation of active flexion motion within the first week or around the end of the first week.

- Short splints for the hand will be used more frequently in the future.

- Proximal pole fractures of the scaphoid should be conservatively treated more frequently.

- Multiple short incisions can replace often used a long S incision in forearm compartment decompression, because in modern times the patient is diagnosed and treated before tissues necrosis and severe involvement of the deep tissues is seldom seen. With multiple shorter incisions, skin grafting is usually unnecessary.

- Elevation of the operated hand after surgery is unnecessary unless the trauma or surgery is extensive or severe hand edema is expected.

REFERENCES

1. Elliot D. Proximal median nerve compressions: anterior interosseous nerve compression - a myth. J Hand Surg Eur 2022;47:540–1.
2. Tang JB. Compression to the anterior interosseous nerve is very rare: compression by the normal tissues surrounding it may not exist. J Hand Surg Eur 2022;47:541–2.
3. Boeckstyns M. My current views on the anterior interosseous nerve syndrome. J Hand Surg Eur 2022;47:542–3.
4. Leblebicioğlu G. Two clinical observations: pronator syndrome in violinists and anterior interosseous nerve syndrome with pure motor loss. J Hand Surg Eur 2022;47:543–5.
5. Upton AR, McComas AJ. The double crush in nerve entrapment syndromes. Lancet 1973;302(7825):359–62.
6. Baba M, Fowler CJ, Jacobs JM, et al. Changes in peripheral nerve fibres distal to a constriction. J Neurol Sci 1982;54:197–208.
7. Dellon AL, Mackinnon SE. Chronic nerve compression model for the double crush hypothesis. Ann Plast Surg 1991;26:259–64.
8. Nemoto K, Matsumoto N, Tazaki K, et al. An experimental study on the "double crush" hypothesis. J Hand Surg Am 1987;12:552–9.
9. Kane PM, Daniels AH, Akelman E. Double crush syndrome. J Am Acad Orthop Surg 2015;23:558–62.
10. Wilbourn AJ, Gilliatt RW. Double-crush syndrome: a critical analysis. Neurology 1997;49:21–9.
11. Osterman AL. The double crush syndrome. Orthop Clin North Am 1988;19:147–55.
12. Bednarik J, Kadanka Z, Vohánka S. Median nerve mononeuropathy in spondylotic cervical myelopathy: Double crush syndrome? J Neurol 1999;246:544–51.
13. Morgan G, Wilbourn AJ. Cervical radiculopathy and coexisting distal entrapment neuropathies: Double-crush syndromes? Neurology 1998;50:78–83.
14. Galarza M, Gazzeri R, Gazzeri G, et al. Cubital tunnel surgery in patients with cervical radiculopathy: double crush syndrome? Neurosurg Rev 2009;32:471–8.

15. Tang JB. Median nerve compression: lacertus syndrome versus superficialis-pronator syndrome. J Hand Surg Eur 2021;46:1017–22.

16. Tang JB. Radial tunnel syndrome: definition, distinction and treatments. J Hand Surg Eur 2020;45: 882–9.

17. Tang JB. Uncommon methods of flexor tendon and tendon-bone repairs and grafting. Hand Clin 2013; 29:215–21.

18. Le Viet D. Flexor tendon lengthening by tenotomy at the musculotendinous junction. Ann Plast Surg 1986;17:239–46.

19. Tang JB. Rehabilitation after flexor tendon repair and others: a safe and efficient protocol. J Hand Surg Eur 2021;46:813–7.

20. Tang JB, Lalonde D, Harhaus L, et al. Flexor tendon repair: recent changes and current methods. J Hand Surg Eur 2022;47:31–9.

21. Tang JB. Recent evolutions in flexor tendon repairs and rehabilitation. J Hand Surg Eur 2018;43:469–73.

22. Wong JK, Peck F. Improving results of flexor tendon repair and rehabilitation. Plast Reconstr Surg 2014; 134:913e–25e.

23. Street J, Nessa L, Logan A, et al. A 4-year study of the use of the short metacarpal cast in the management of metacarpal shaft fractures. J Hand Surg Eur 2021;46:936–40.

24. Gellman H, Caputo RJ, Carter V, et al. Comparison of short and long thumb-spica casts for non-displaced fractures of the carpal scaphoid. J Bone Joint Surg Am 1989;71:354–7.

25. Grewal R, Lutz K, MacDermid JC, et al. proximal pole scaphoid fractures: a computed tomographic assessment of outcomes. J Hand Surg Am 2016; 41:54–8.

26. Dias JJ, Ring D, Grewal R, et al. Acute scaphoid fractures: making decisions for treating a troublesome bone. J Hand Surg Eur 2022;47:73–9.

27. Johnson NA, Dias JJ. Scaphoid waist fracture displacement within 2 mm and most proximal pole fractures do not need surgical treatment. J Hand Surg Eur 2021;46:1023–6.

28. Suh N, Grewal R. Controversies and best practices for acute scaphoid fracture management. J Hand Surg Eur 2018;43:4–12.

29. Tang JB. On the safe position for hand immobilization. J Hand Surg Eur 2019;44:993–5.

Moving?

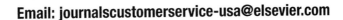

Make sure your subscription moves with you!

To notify us of your new address, find your **Clinics Account Number** (located on your mailing label above your name), and contact customer service at:

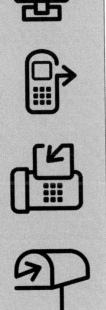

Email: journalscustomerservice-usa@elsevier.com

800-654-2452 (subscribers in the U.S. & Canada)
314-447-8871 (subscribers outside of the U.S. & Canada)

Fax number: 314-447-8029

Elsevier Health Sciences Division
Subscription Customer Service
3251 Riverport Lane
Maryland Heights, MO 63043

*To ensure uninterrupted delivery of your subscription, please notify us at least 4 weeks in advance of move.

Printed and bound by CPI Group (UK) Ltd, Croydon, CR0 4YY

08/05/2025

01864715-0008